The Diet Doctors

Doctors

Inside and Out

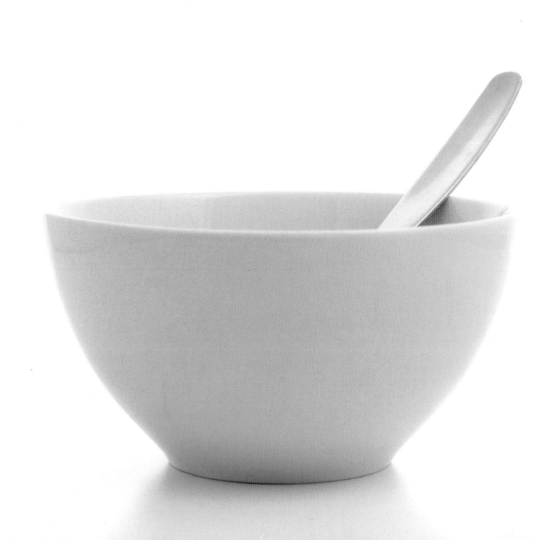

The Diet Doctors

Inside and Out

The Full Body Makeover Plan That Gets Results

Dr Wendy Denning and Vicki Edgson

Vermilion

1 3 5 7 9 10 8 6 4 2

First published in the United Kingdom in 2006 by Vermilion,
an imprint of Ebury Publishing
Random House UK Ltd.
Random House
20 Vauxhall Bridge Road
London SW1V 2SA

Random House Australia (Pty) Limited
20 Alfred Street, Milsons Point, Sydney,
New South Wales 2061, Australia

Random House New Zealand Limited
18 Poland Road, Glenfield,
Auckland 10, New Zealand

Random House (Pty) Limited
Isle of Houghton, Corner Boundary Road & Carse O'Gowrie,
Houghton, 2198 South Africa

Random House UK Limited Reg. No. 954009
www.randomhouse.co.uk
Papers used by Vermilion are natural, recyclable products made from wood grown in sustainable forests.

A CIP catalogue record is available for this book from the British Library.

ISBN: 0091910501

Project managed and designed by Emma Marriott and
Dan Newman/Perfect Books Ltd

Printed and bound in Italy by Graphicom SRL

Although every effort has been made to ensure the contents of this book are accurate, it must not be treated as a substitute for qualified medical advice. Always consult a medical practitioner. Neither the author nor the publisher can be held responsible for any loss or claim arising out of the use, or misuse, of the information and suggestions contained in this book, or the failure to take medical advice.

Supplement Recommendations

Please note that dosages for supplements have not been given because they will vary from person to person according to size, shape and other needs. If you are taking other medication, it is advisable to check with your doctor before taking any herbal remedies. In all cases, it is also wise to be under the care of a trained nutritionist or doctor who specialises in nutritional medicine to give you an expert view.

DEDICATION

To my mother who made me aware of the power of
food for good health and who is always one supplement
ahead of me; and to my father who believed that a good
education is critical and made sure I got one – Dr Wendy

I dedicate this book to Andrew, who creatively
challenges my every word, thought and belief – Vicki

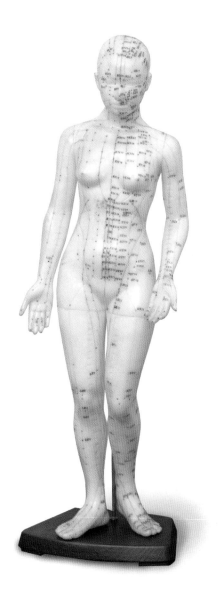

Contents

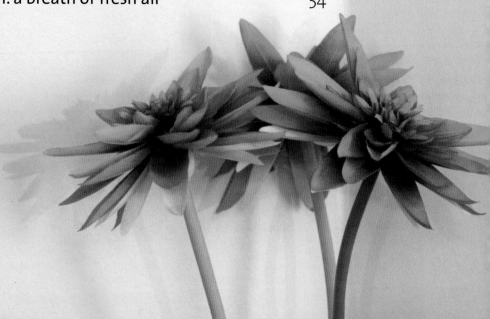

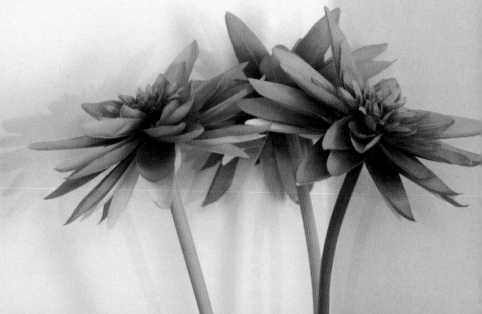

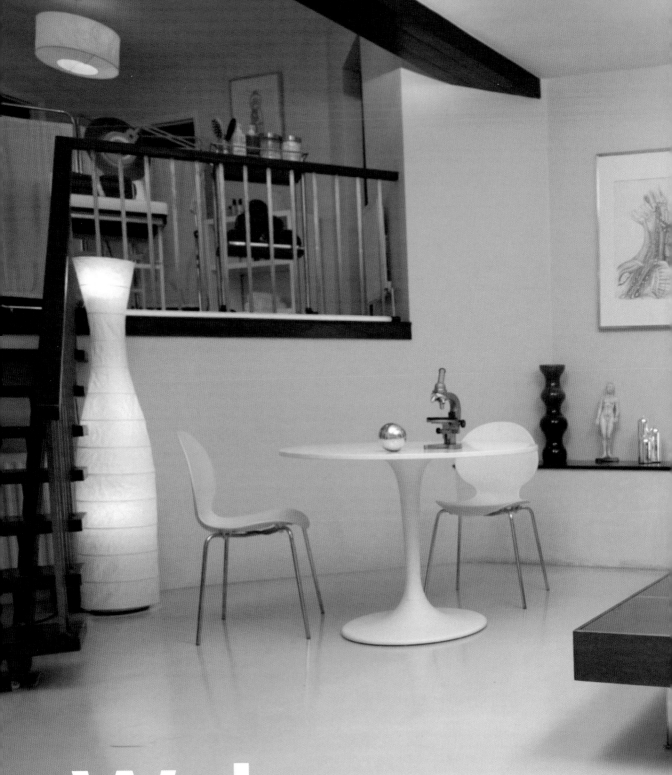

Welcome...

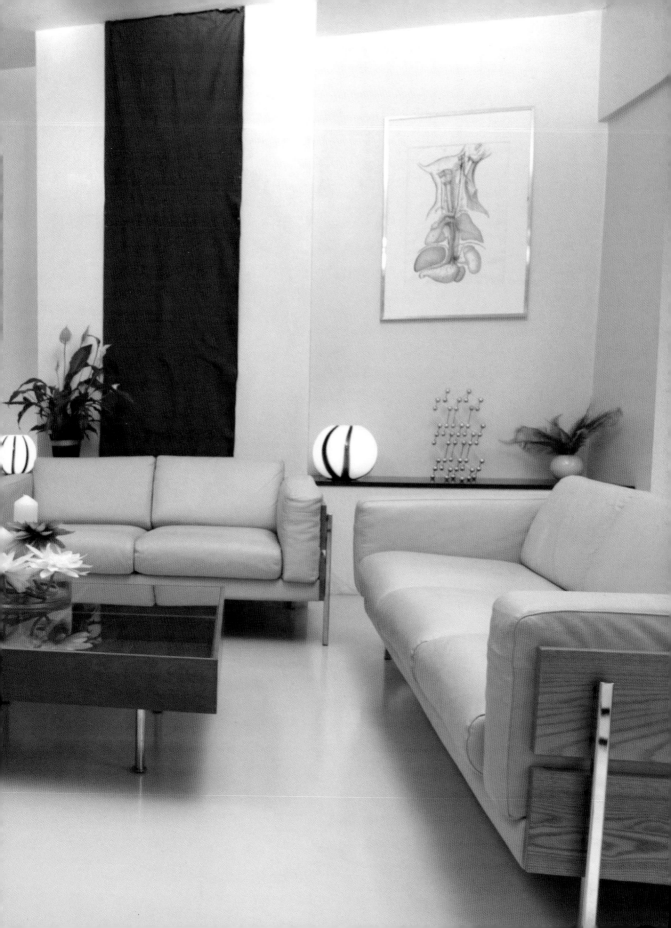

Introduction

The inspiration for this book comes from 30 years of collective practice as a doctor and nutritionist, during which time we have helped many patients to lose weight and improve their multitude of health problems. With simple changes to their diet and lifestyle, they have watched the pounds drop off and their health problems disappear.

Our collective wisdom which we share with you in this book comes from our individual training in conventional medicine, nutrition and traditional Chinese medicine, which we have simplified to make it more accessible for you. We give you the tools to drop the excess pounds and, at the same time, alleviate common health problems that frequently arise from years of improper eating, drinking, smoking and lack of exercise.

Six out of ten people in Britain are now overweight or obese

Did you realise that in this country we consume over one billion pounds' worth of ready-made meals per year and spend three billion on fast foods? And yet, at the same time, we also spend over two million pounds on diet products? Or that six out of ten people are now overweight or obese? Clearly these eating patterns are not making us thinner.

Did you also realise that diabetes is now the third largest killer after heart disease and cancers, and that, according to the World Health Organisation, this is directly attributable to obesity, diet and lifestyles? So our current eating patterns are not making us healthy either.

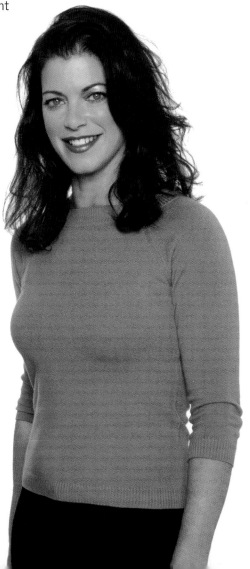

There's no getting away from it: if you're overweight, you should expect to feel tired and lethargic, to suffer from digestive problems and to have aching joints and back because your body has to take the strain of an extra load. Many ailments are a result of being overweight and most conditions included in this book are directly related to excess weight. A pill may take away the pain and alleviate some of the symptoms, but it won't get rid of the root of the problem. In this book we're going to give you the solutions to the problem – we'll give you the tools to enable you to formulate your own tailor-made diet plan.

Your body is constantly talking to you. It's sending you messages right now, but are you listening? In the first part of the book, we're going to teach you to recognise the signals. Start to read them properly and you can help your body cure itself. So whether you've got permanent goose bumps on the back of your arms, a swollen tongue, or dry and lifeless hair, by the end of the first section of the book you'll know how to recognise what these signs mean, what your body doesn't like and what it needs more of.

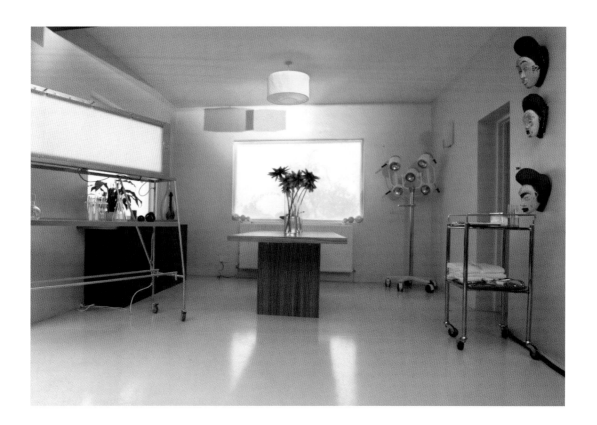

To understand why your body is telling you all this, you need to know how it works, so we explain the vital systems, and suggest simple diagnostic tests that you can do at home. You'll begin to realise that our bodies are unique and each of us has different food requirements. There's no point in eating a chicken sandwich for lunch if you've got an intolerance to wheat, or eating a lot of salad and raw vegetables if you're not able to digest them. As you read this book, and try some of the tests, you'll begin to recognise what YOUR body needs.

The good news is that no matter how unfit or overweight you are, or how you've abused your body in the past, it is extremely forgiving. It has an amazing capacity to repair and rejuvenate itself very quickly, given what it needs. Even organs like the liver, which generally bears the load from too much fatty food, alcohol and sugar, can recover completely. It's never too late to make a difference and if you change your diet and lifestyle now, your body will feel the benefits immediately.

The second half of the book will teach you the fundamentals about food and how it works in your body, providing you with an Eating for Life food programme. This programme will balance your blood sugar, give you more energy, and help you lose the extra pounds and smooth out those mood swings. It will help the digestive system work as effectively as possible which we believe is a fundamental key to good health. Finally, rather than limiting the foods that you can eat, this programme will do the opposite, introducing you to foods you may never have heard of and telling you how to prepare them in easy, delicious recipes.

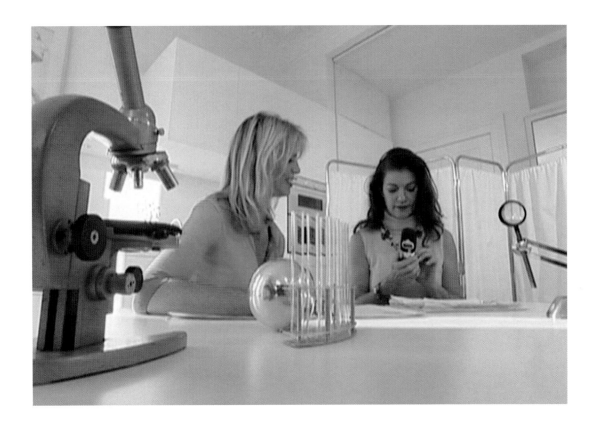

There is another part to this health and weight loss equation which is too often ignored in our busy lives – exercise. Getting moving is vital and it doesn't have to involve a gym membership. You simply have to use the opportunities in your day to get moving; be that climbing the stairs rather than using the escalator, getting off the bus one stop earlier, taking regular breaks from your desk, or taking yourself for a 30 minute brisk walk four times a week.

We hope that you enjoy reading this book and that it inspires you to reclaim and maintain your health by engaging with your body, taking responsibility for it and making the changes that you need to experience vibrant health.

Your body can recover from the damage you've inflicted on it – it's never too late to change your diet and lifestyle

introduction

What should I weigh?

Ask any two people with the same height and frame what their ideal weight would be and you're guaranteed to get a different answer. There is no ideal specific weight for any one person, that figure will be down to your own personal choice. However, we can provide you with an ideal weight range and there are three different ways for you to obtain this range.

The Body Mass Index

The Body Mass Index is probably the most widely used method currently. It uses an equation that takes height and weight into consideration, making it more precise than relying on scales alone. The equation is:

$$\frac{\text{weight in kilograms}}{\text{height in metres x height in metres}}$$

For example, if your weight is 80kg and your height is 1.8m then your BMI will be 80 divided by 1.8 x 1.8 = **24**. To convert imperial measurements to metric, see page 219.

BMI chart

Weight	BMI
Normal weight	20-25
Overweight	25-30
Seriously overweight/Obese	30-40
Dangerously overweight/Obese	40+

For ideal body weight you need to be 25 or less. In fact, if your BMI is higher than 27 it increases your risk for every single condition outlined in this book and, on top of that, increases the risk of breast, colon, endometrial, kidney and oesophageal cancer. With a BMI of 30 or more you are considered to be obese and, as your level rises, so your risk goes up. There is also evidence linking obesity to cancer of the pancreas, uterus, prostate and ovary.

So BMI is very useful but, like anything, it has its limitations. It does not take into account body fat and muscle ratios, meaning that an athlete and a desk worker who never exercises can have similar BMIs. This is because fat weighs less than non-fat lean muscle. Furthermore, as you age the proportion of lean muscle to body fat (which is less dense) increases. This is an important fact to grasp because as you lose weight and start exercising you may find that your clothes are looser but the scales aren't budging. This is where measuring on specialised scales and doing body measurements may be helpful, because you may be replacing fat for muscle.

Lean Body Mass

There are now scales available that measure your body fat as a percentage of your total weight. Whilst trying to lose weight you also want to make sure that you are losing fat, and converting fat into muscle. So if these scales show you are not losing weight, but your body fat percentage is going down, that is good progress. If you want a quick guide to do at home without buying the scales, do the pinch test.

The pinch test involves pinching the fleshy skin at the back of your upper arm between your thumb and index finger. If your finger and thumb are more than 2cm or ¾ inch apart when you squeeze then you are probably overweight. The scales may be more accurate and make it easier to assess progress.

Here is the body fat percentage you should be aiming for at a particular age.

Age	Males	Females
10-30	10-18%	20-25%
31-40	13-19%	21-27%
41-50	14-20%	22-28%
51-60	16-20%	22-30%
60+	17-21%	22-31%

Waist Circumference

The simplest test for being overweight is to measure your waist circumference. A recent study has shown that it is a good predictor of health problems since abdominal obesity is associated with fat on the main organs (including the liver and heart) and contributes to cardiovascular disease and diabetes.

A waist circumference of more than 102cm (40in) for men and 88cm (35in) for women is associated with increased risk of health problems. This is because this measurement is closely linked to the Metabolic Syndrome (see page 98).

Ideally you should do all three tests in order to calculate most accurately what your target weight should be. However, each test will give you a good idea of how much weight you need to lose.

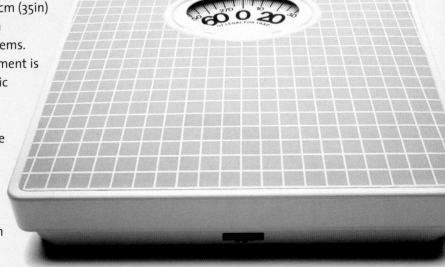

What yo is trying tell you

Your body is constantly talking to you and drawing your attention to its needs. There are many signs that you yourself can observe – and learning to recognise them is a good starting point for diagnosis. In this chapter we provide you with some guides to those signals and offer some simple remedies for immediate action. The next section 'How Your Body Works' looks at the bigger picture and explains in depth what is going on behind the scenes.

ur body
to

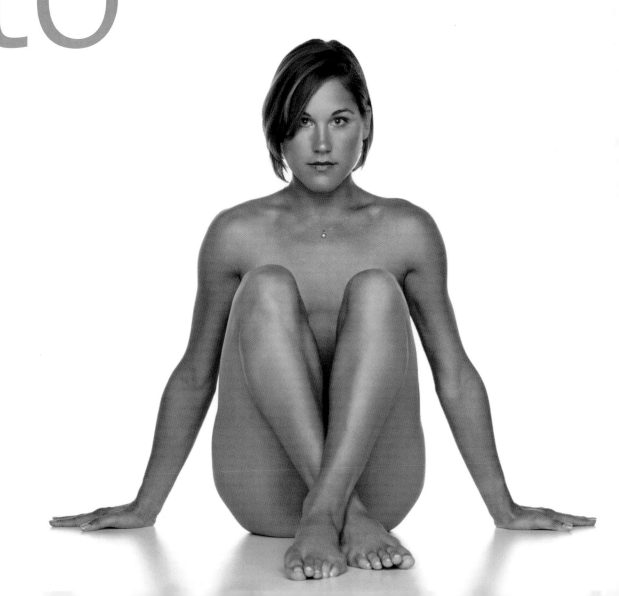

The tongue

Until quite recently, patients' tongues were examined by doctors as a matter of routine – the idea being that this would provide a good indicator of their state of health. Sadly, the practice is less common now, though still widely used for diagnosis in Chinese and Ayurvedic medicine, with excellent benefits.

Our tongues change everyday but it's incredible just how much the general condition of your tongue can be transformed by following a good eating plan. A large, puffy and pale tongue can become smaller and pinker in a just a few weeks. It's a general but fantastically useful diagnostic tool and if you can learn to read the signals displayed in your tongue it will become a lifelong reference point for general health.

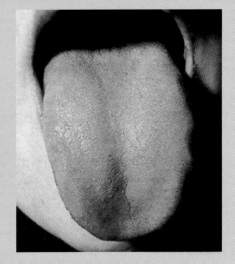

When you examine your tongue, it is important to do so in as bright a light as possible. Wait some time after eating, drinking or taking medicine, which may colour the tongue coating. Scraping the tongue may remove valuable information, so examine it before doing so.

There are three things to look at when examining the tongue: its shape/size, its colour and its coating. The normal tongue (right) is salmon pink/light red, with a thin, white, moist coating, and is smooth with no cracks.

Examining your tongue

Dr Wendy says: 'Different areas of the tongue are linked to several key systems of the body and so can give us valuable clues to the state of our health. I have used my training in traditional Chinese medicine to provide a few clues which can be useful in the assessment of health.'

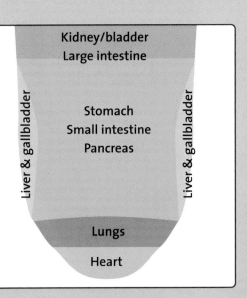

Kidney/bladder
Large intestine

Liver & gallbladder

Stomach
Small intestine
Pancreas

Liver & gallbladder

Lungs

Heart

Colour

✚ Pale

A pale tongue (top right) points to a state of deficiency in the body – a lack of vitamins, minerals and/or protein, and/or hormones and neurotransmitters. Typical symptoms include fatigue and lethargy, cold hands and feet, a tendency to feel the cold, anaemia or iron deficiency, underactive thyroid, dizziness, shortness of breath, pale complexion, frequent urination and lack of libido.

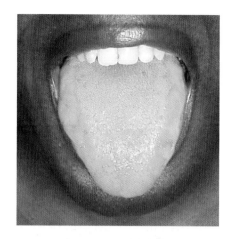

✚ Red

A red tongue (middle right) may point to acute fever, generally feeling hot more than cold, sweating easily, thirst, tendency to constipation (or firmer stools than normal), irritability, bad temper and/or anger, skin problems, night sweats, excess alcohol or coffee consumption, taking drugs (prescribed or not), hives or headaches.

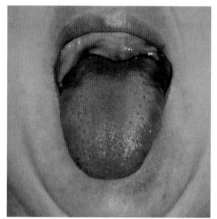

✚ A red tip

This may indicate stress, insomnia or a tendency to be upset or depressed – you may have PMT or be mildly irritable. (A red tip can also be seen in the top photo on page 21.)

✚ Purple

A purple tongue (bottom right) generally equates to poor circulation of blood or other fluids in the body, with corresponding symptoms. These include menstrual cramps, endometriosis, fibroids, breast cysts, pain in a specific area of the body such as back ache, cold arms and legs, headaches, dull skin and varicose veins. It may also be associated with muscle spasms.

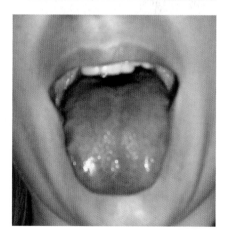

The tongue is a fantastically useful diagnostic tool

tongue

The general condition of your tongue can be transformed in just a few weeks by following a good eating plan

Shape/size

✚ Swollen

A swollen tongue is generally associated with a problem in the digestive system, unless it is just swollen on the sides, in which case it signifies a problem with the liver. Symptoms vary according to the nature of the swelling.

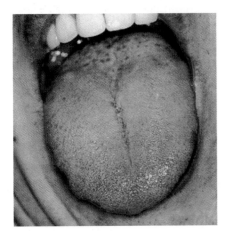

Swollen and pale: tendency to feeling cold, and can also indicate poor digestion, spontaneous sweating at rest, fatigue, bloating and feeling heavy in the legs.

Swollen and red: (left) tendency to being irritable, angry and thirsty, and can indicate headaches, skin problems and maybe too much coffee, alcohol and/or drug consumption in the face of a poor underlying digestive system.

Swelling to the sides of the tongue: usually indicates a problem with the liver or gallbladder. Most often it will mean the liver is being overworked to some degree.

✚ Teeth marks to sides of tongue

Teeth marks on both sides of the tongue (a mild case can be seen above) usually accompany a swollen tongue. The teeth press against the tongue because it has become too big for the mouth, causing these indentations. This is usually caused by a poor digestive system, where the body is not getting enough nutrition from food, or by too little sleep the previous night. Associated symptoms include poor digestion, gas and bloating, loose stools (a common feature of a poor digestive system), body bruising easily – due to lack of vitamin C and other nutrients that make the blood vessels strong – fatigue and shortness of breath.

Coating

The coating is one of the most important signs to read, so don't run to the bathroom and scrub your tongue before you have truly analysed its condition. If your tongue does not have a thin white coating (top right), then you have a problem. Too much coating, and you have a sluggish system, depending on where the coating is; too little coating, and you have too much heat in your system, leading to other problems.

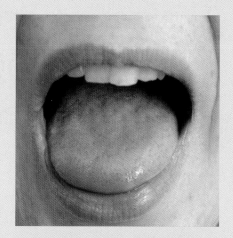

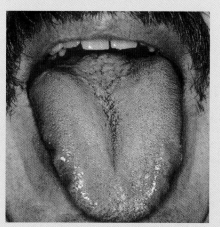

✚ Thick white coating

This may be associated with a viral illness, e.g. a cold, fatigue, lethargy, feeling cold, heavy feelings in arms and legs and swollen ankles.

A thick white coating at the back of the tongue (bottom right) could indicate poor digestion and lack of beneficial bacteria.

✚ Brown coating

This is linked to constipation, smoking and excess coffee intake.

✚ Yellow coating

A yellow coating is usually seen with a red tongue, indicating a tendency to be overheated in the body and being irritable, angry or stressed.

✚ Black coating

This is more common than you think and can be quite an alarming sight. It can be caused by high fever from dehydration, infectious diseases, digestive problems, fungus infection as well as long term use of antibiotics.

✚ Peeling

A peeling tongue can indicate a dry mouth and throat, febrile illness, overindulgence in spicy food, discomfort in upper abdomen (e.g. heartburn/lack of stomach acid), nausea and poor absorption of food – often due to a deficiency in B vitamins.

tongue

Skin

Dr Wendy says: 'When you greet a friend there are two things you automatically register about that person: the skin and the eyes. The health of your body is reflected in the skin and, for this reason, both Vicki and I use the skin as one of our first diagnostic tools. Even before the patient has sat down we have already gathered a huge amount of information about that person's health.'

The skin is directly or indirectly linked to almost every organ in the book. It is also a major organ of elimination in the body (the others being the colon, the kidney and the lungs). So, if those organs are struggling to get rid of waste and toxins, then more will show up on the skin in the form of oiliness, excess sweating, and rashes.

The most obvious signs to look out for are colour, texture (dry or oily), lines, stretch marks, and the presence of any inflammation such as rashes.

Colour

The skin contains varying levels of pigment that give it its particular colour. Black and Asian skin is more likely to develop extra pigmentation in areas of scarring and so you need to protect it against acne and injury. Other indicators which are sometimes more apparent on white skin are:

✛ **Pale**

You could be anaemic, have low iron or an underactive thyroid.

✛ **Red**

You could be angry, just have exercised, be suffering with a fever or be drinking too much coffee and alcohol. You could be more prone to developing arthritic symptoms due to a generalised degree of inflammation in the body as well as possibly suffering hormone imbalances.

✛ **Yellow**

You may be jaundiced and have a problem with your liver.

✛ **Grey**

You may be a smoker, have been pushing the body too hard, suffering with a sluggish liver or could be suffering with an underlying cardiovascular disease or other serious illness.

Texture

Dry skin

Dry skin lacks oils and moisture and is caused by a deficient intake of water and essential fatty acids, omega-3, 6 and 9. It is more common with fair-skinned people because black skin naturally has more oil in it. It can be associated with deficiencies in vitamin A (as can many skin problems) and the B vitamins, and can be aggravated by drinking too much coffee, tea and alcohol, all of which dehydrate you.

It is also closely related to our hormones so it can be associated with the menopause and an underactive thyroid in women, and aging in men. It can also be seen in chronic inflammatory skin conditions, such as eczema and dermatitis. And as we age, our skin generally tends to get drier, giving our appearance a more aged look. It is amazing how much younger you can look if you just reduce your coffee and tea intake and drink more water. Why do you think that models drink eight glasses of pure water per day when they are working?

Oily skin

The great advantage of oily skin is that it ages at a slower rate than other skin types. It is produced by sebaceous glands producing more oil than the skin needs. It is common in teenagers and can occur when stressed, pregnant and in the menopause because of hormone imbalances. There is a genetic influence but it can also be brought on by the birth control pill, your diet and use of cosmetics. It can be associated with a diet high in salt, sugar and saturated fats, and even a slight deficiency of vitamin B2 can cause this; so keep up your intake of wholegrains and beans.

Many people have skin that is oily in certain areas and dry or normal in others, a condition known as combination skin. For this it helps to reduce your intake of salt, sugar and saturated fats and take lots of water to help detoxify the body .

Lines on the face

The commonest causes of lines are exposure to sunlight, dry skin, smoking, aging due to loss of hormones (not so apparent if these are replaced), and persistent facial expressions. Black skin has a little more oil and, because of its darker skin pigment, is more protected from the sun's aging effects and less likely to wrinkle.

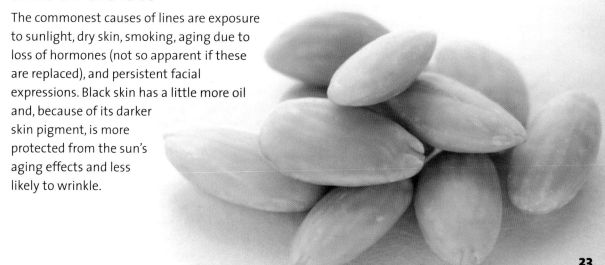

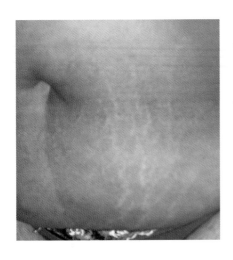

Stretch marks

These are usually associated with pregnancy, but can often be caused by rapid weight gain. They're also more likely when your diet is low in fruit and vegetables and therefore vitamin C, which is needed to produce elastin and collagen (which is important for the skin's condition). Low levels of zinc are a factor here too, zinc being important for the healing of wounds.

They are more apparent in black and asian women, because of the skin's propensity to develop extra pigmentation in areas of scarring.

With stretch marks, prevention is definitely better than the cure as, once you have them, they will fade over time but not necessarily disappear.

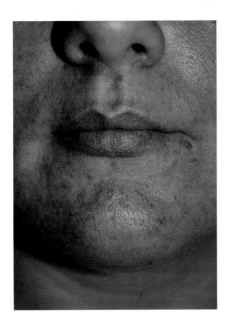

Skin rashes

If you have just developed a skin rash, the first thing to consider is whether you have recently started a new medication or changed one. Following this, you should think about what chemicals you have in your home, have been exposed to or used on your skin. Alternatively, of course, you may have developed a skin infection such as chicken pox.

If the answer to all of these things is no, it could be that your liver is causing the problem. Remember that the skin eliminates toxic waste. So if the liver – the major organ of detoxification – is overloaded, more will be excreted out through the skin. Cleaning up your liver is therefore critical. For more advice, see the section on skin (page 114-121).

QUICK TIP: If you are suffering with permanent goose bumps on your arms in hot and cold weather then you are suffering with a condition known as hyperfollicular keratitis. Take more omega-3 and 6, both in your diet and with supplements, and this condition should disappear in 1-3 months.

Healthy skin action plan

In general terms, most people don't realise how much the skin depends for its condition on them drinking lots of water, eating a good diet and keeping up levels of essential vitamins and minerals. You could start your own beauty regime here and now – no need to book a plastic surgeon!

+ Increase your water intake to eight glasses of water per day.

+ Stop smoking.

+ Protect your skin when you go out in the sunlight with a hat and sunscreen.

+ Look after your digestive system – for further information on this see the section on digestion (pages 60-83).

+ Look after your liver – by cutting down on your alcohol and drug use.

+ Check for food intolerances (see page 69).

+ Eat a diet with 6 to 8 helpings of vegetables and fruit per day – the best antioxidants which will limit ageing in the skin.

+ Keep up your intake of the essential fatty acids by eating more oily fish such as salmon, sardines, mackerel and pumpkin and sunflower seeds.

+ Keep up your intake of zinc with turkey, eggs, almonds, peas.

+ Reduce your saturated fat intake.

See a nutritionist, or a doctor if you think you may have more serious health concerns.

Supplements for the skin

+ Good multivitamin and mineral
+ Flaxseed oil – 2 tablespoons – or omega-3 fish oil supplement
+ Oil of evening primrose
+ Zinc
+ Aloe vera

Healthy skin depends on drinking plenty of water

skin

Eyes

Not only are eyes the window to the soul, but they're also the window to much of what is going on in different parts of the body, particularly the liver.

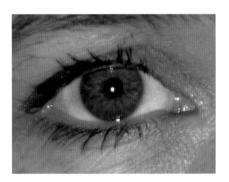

Have you ever looked at your eyes in the mirror the morning after a particularly heavy night out? Are they bloodshot, with a dull haze over the cornea? A sharp contrast to clear, bright, sparkling eyes, which usually indicate good health and abundant energy.

One major contributor to eye problems is a poor diet. A deficiency of just one vitamin can lead to various eye conditions.

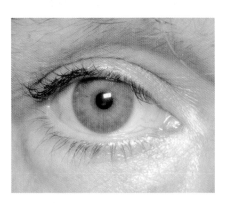

Yellow eyes

This may indicate a problem with your liver or gallbladder, with a build up of bilirubin and you should see your doctor. However the most common cause of slightly yellow eyes is a condition called Gilbert's syndrome, which occurs in 5–10 per cent of people. Due to an inherited enzyme deficiency in the liver, bilirubin builds up in the liver particularly when the person is fasting or stressed. If this is you, take milk thistle (a liver supporting herb) when you are stressed.

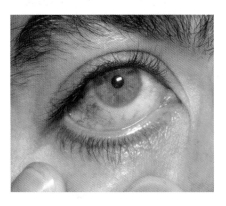

Bloodshot eyes

This happens when the small blood vessels on the surface of the eye become inflamed and congested with blood. This can be caused by eyestrain, fatigue and too much alcohol. It can also be due to a deficiency of vitamins B2 and B6 and certain amino acids that come from protein in the diet. Try getting more sleep, reducing your alcohol intake and spending fewer hours at the computer. If that doesn't do the trick, then take a B-complex vitamin, milk thistle and more protein.

Dark circles under the eyes

These are very often due to lack of sleep, but they may also run in families or indicate a problem with your digestive system, particularly with the colon or an overloaded liver. Check for food intolerances (see page 69), parasites in the bowel, constipation (see page 64) and a sluggish liver(see page 80), but do make sure you are getting enough sleep first!

Bags under the eyes

Bags (right) may occur at any age but is more common with age as the skin loses some of its elasticity and the local muscles their tone, so fluids and fat accumulate. In all people it can be associated with excess salt intake, lack of sleep, smoking and food sensitivities. In older people it can also be due to a sluggish thyroid (see page 90) or a kidney problem (see urine test for protein page 35). So reduce your salt intake, get more sleep, stop smoking and stop drinking fluids before you go to bed. Getting checked for food sensitivities can be helpful as can checking with your doctor to rule out more serious issues.

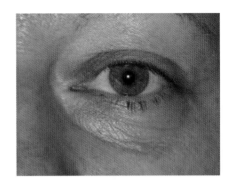

Poor night vision

This may indicate a deficiency in vitamin A or beta carotene, in which case you should eat more carrots or drink freshly-made carrot juice. Adding a supplement may also be helpful.

Dry eyes

Naturally enough, eyes get dry when the tear ducts don't produce enough tears to keep them moist. This is more common in women, particularly after the menopause. It happens quite commonly in contact lens wearers, and people who stare at a computer screen all day. It may also be due to deficiencies in omega-3 and 6 essential fatty acids (see page 137), a sluggish thyroid (see page 90), a side effect of drugs or a complication of a condition such as rheumatoid arthritis (see page 127). Always make sure you are taking enough vitamin A in your diet and with supplements. If you suspect that your dry eyes could be due to a prescription drug, check with your doctor to see if there is an alternative. Traditional Chinese medicine is often very useful for this condition.

Itching eyes

This may be due to hay fever, allergies to cosmetics, food and chemicals, or a vitamin B deficiency. Make sure you are taking enough B vitamins in your diet, and add a supplement if you are stressed, as B vitamins get used up very quickly under such pressure.

Bulging eyes

This can be caused by an overactive thyroid. Get this checked by your doctor.

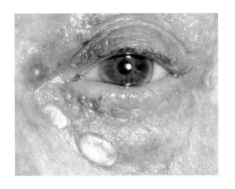

Yellow spots under the eyes

These (right) may be caused by a thyroid problem (see page 90) or an elevated level of cholesterol in your blood (see page 48). Visit your doctor and get both possibilities checked.

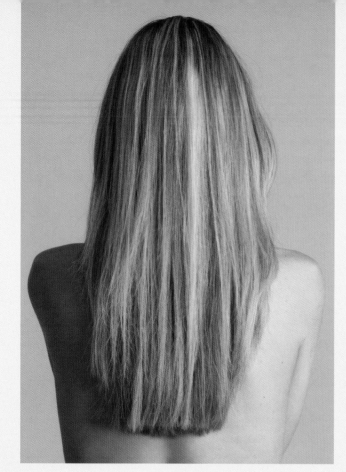

Hair

Hair can be a surprisingly good indicator of your overall good health – a healthy person's hair is reflected in a shiny, thick head of hair. This is because hair, which is made of protein, keratin and minerals, depends for its condition on the amount of nutrients it is receiving from the scalp. So a good diet and good digestive system are essential.

Hair grows in a cyclical fashion, a growth phase followed by a resting phase. After the resting phase, the hair is shed and the cycle repeats itself. It is normal to lose 50–100 hairs every day. Sadly, from the age of about 20 onwards, hair starts to thin gradually.

Excess body hair

How much body hair a person likes is a matter of personal preference although excess body hair is usually more of a concern for women than men. In the main, it's your genes that determine how much hair you have, but excess body hair on women can also be caused by a hormone imbalance in the body, such as with polycystic ovary syndrome (see page 87) where excessive androgens (male sex hormones) are produced by the body.

Excessive hair can also be an age-related problem – some women develop excess body hair as they get older because the hair follicles become more sensitive to androgens. The same can apply to men, many of whom often find hair growing from their ears and nose as they age. It can also be a side-effect of certain drugs, such as cortisone. If you suspect this or polycystic ovary syndrome, then see your doctor for diagnosis.

If you have polycystic ovary syndrome then reducing your weight and following the polycystic ovary action plan (see page 88) is crucial. Saw palmetto (a herb used in men with prostate problems) can also be of benefit, as can medication from your doctor.

Thinning hair

This happens in both men and women, the pattern determined by genes and hormones. If men lose enough hair, they become bald. Women on the other hand will almost never go bald (unless they are on chemotherapy or radiotherapy), but their hair tends to thin with age, with the loss more generalised over the scalp. Hair loss may be brought on sooner, however, by childbirth, or a severe emotional shock such as divorce or bereavement. Other factors include stress, a poor diet, lack of iron, thyroid disease and sudden weight loss.

Dry hair

Dry hair may be associated with inadequate protein intake, essential fatty acid deficiency, thyroid disease and the menopause. It can also be caused by the chemicals you use on your hair.

Greying hair

Greying hair is most commonly associated with aging; pigment cells are lost in the hair and skin as we age. It is usually genetically predetermined, but can occasionally be caused by an auto-immune condition where the body perceives the pigment cells in the hair as foreign and attacks them. It can also be brought on abruptly by a major shock such as a bereavement, or by chronic anaemia and thyroid problems. If the last two apply to you, your doctor can help.

Healthy hair action plan

If you want to improve the condition of your hair, then you could try the following suggestions. Start with the first five, and then add in the others if necessary.

+ Eat enough protein.

+ Chew your food well so that you absorb all its nutrients.

+ Make sure you are not mineral deficient (see page 39) and correct any deficiencies particularly of iron, zinc and selenium (because they boost the thyroid).

+ Take a good multivitamin and mineral specifically designed for the hair.

+ Take flaxseed oil to maintain levels of omega-3 and 6.

+ Take silica or horsetail, which helps to keep the hair looking shiny and sleek.

+ Eat seaweed – one of the richest sources of minerals.

+ Try relaxation techniques if you're stressed (stress will reduce blood circulation to your scalp).

+ Get a scalp massage to improve blood supply to your head.

hair

Nails

Nails provide a protective covering to the ends of toes and fingers, and are often seen as a symbol of beauty. They are in the skin family, so anything that affects the skin will often affect the nails as well. Checking your nails can be a good way to determine if you have nutritional deficiencies or other health issues.

The nail bed is the skin on which the nails grow. Composed mainly of keratin (which is a protein), a fingernail takes about four months to grow out, and a toenail at least six months. The rate of growth can be slowed down by a fungal infection of the nails and general nutritional deficiency, particularly of protein. So if your nails are growing slowly and are discoloured, suspect a fungal infection; and if they're not discoloured, then suspect a nutritional deficiency.

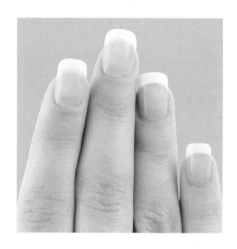

In fact, anything that impairs the body's absorption and use of proteins for tissue repair can cause abnormal growth, including acute or chronic illness, poor stomach acid and food intolerances. Good nail growth is also heavily dependent on having the right vitamins, minerals and essential fatty acids (omega-3 and 6), so any deficiencies here will show up very quickly.

Healthy nail beds are pink, and normal nails are white with no pits, white spots, cracks or ridges. Deviations from this ideal can be caused by a whole range of factors.

Discoloured nails

There may be underlying causes in the body, e.g. diabetes, stress, prolonged illness, food intolerances, lack of friendly bacteria (lactobacilli) causing a fungal infection. Or the discoloration may be due to the use of nicotine, or the prolonged use of nail polish and removers.

Brittle nails

This can be caused by iron deficiency, a lack of vitamin A, calcium and essential fatty acids, problems with the thyroid, kidneys or circulation, or simply aging – nails lose their moisture as we age.

Nutritional deficiencies often have visible effects on the nails

White spots

These are associated with zinc and/or calcium deficiency.

Ridges

Horizontal ridges (top right) may be caused by injury, thyroid problems, severe stress (either physical or psychological) or vitamin B deficiency.

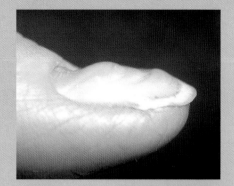

Vertical ridges (middle right) may be caused by poor absorption of nutrients, poor general health, iron deficiency or a kidney disorder.

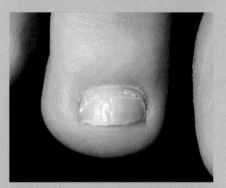

Cracking/peeling nails:

These may be due to lack of vitamin A, calcium, silica and other minerals, insufficient stomach acid and protein.

Red skin around the cuticles

This could be due to insufficient essential fatty acids (omega-3 and 6).

Pitted nails:

These may be caused by psoriasis, or a deficiency of vitamin C, folic acid and protein.

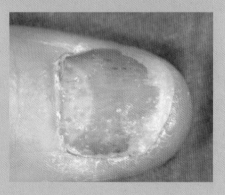

Thick nails

These are associated with poor circulation, thyroid disease or a fungal infection (bottom right). Fungal nail treatments can be hard to treat so early intervention is important. Start with local treatments unless it is very severe. These should include cutting the nail very short and applying tea tree oil or a bandage soaked in vinegar daily. If these don't work then see your doctor for drug treatment.

Spoon-shaped nails

These may be caused by deficiency of iron or vitamin B2.

Pale nail beds

The most common cause is anaemia.

Deep blue nail beds

These may be due to a chronic lung condition, e.g. emphysema, or cyanotic congenital heart disease.

nails

Of course household chemicals or solvents can have a damaging effect on nails. If you repeatedly immerse your hands in water that contains bleaches and soaps, your nails will split, so wear rubber gloves. If you wear nail polish, use a base coat underneath it to stop yellow discoloration. Use nail polish removers as little as possible as they contain solvents that leach the fat from the nails, leaving them brittle. They are also extremely toxic and are absorbed through the skin. Finally, the use of artificial nails has been known to contribute to fungal infections of the fingernails.

Strong nails action plan

+ Eat plenty of good quality vegetable and fish protein – this will help make the keratin strong.

+ Eat more seeds and nuts for essential fatty acids, zinc and protein.

+ Eat 6 to 8 helpings of vegetables and fruit per day.

+ Drink fresh carrot juice daily as it is high in vitamin C and beta carotene, which converts to vitamin A in the body.

+ Eat more cabbage, broccoli, cheese and milk to boost calcium.

+ Increase zinc levels – in oysters, almonds, lamb, haddock and eggs, or by taking a zinc picolinate or food state supplement.

+ Keep your iron levels up through your diet and with supplements if necessary.

+ Take a seaweed or kelp supplement if you have a sluggish thyroid or you want to strengthen the nails, as it is rich in zinc and iodine.

+ Take silica – a highly effective supplement to strengthen your nails.

+ Take hemp seed oil as it provides omega-3 and 6 fatty acids, so is helpful for weak and brittle nails.

If these simple measures don't improve your nails, then consult a nutritional therapist first. If you think you have a more serious problem, then see your doctor.

Eat 6 to 8 portions of fresh fruit and vegetables to strengthen your nails

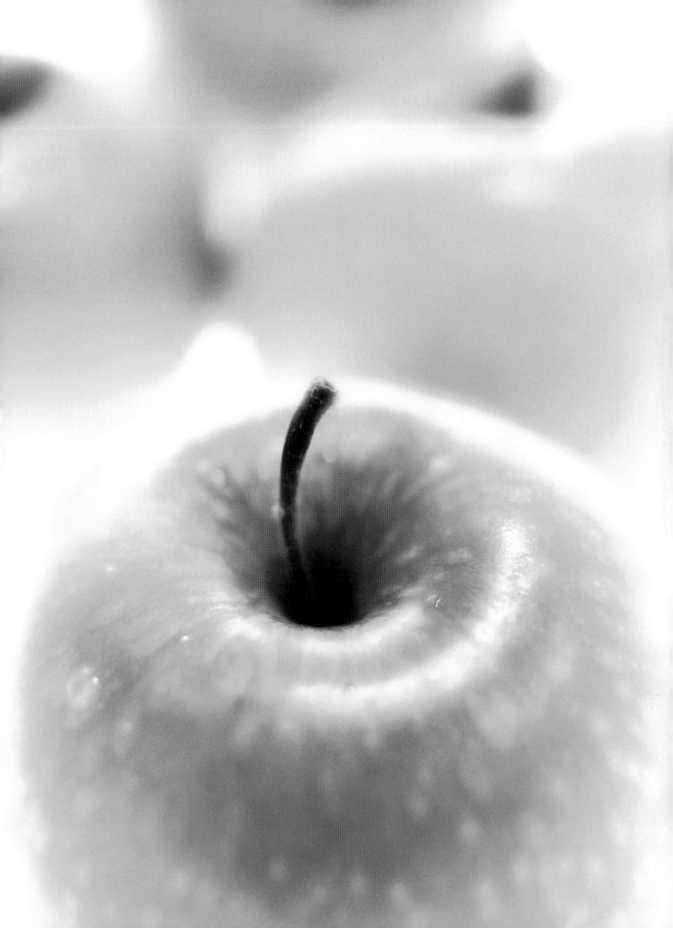

How often do you take a look in the toilet bowl? Like your tongue, the appearance of your stools and urine can change from one day to the next but the general condition can give us a lot of information about how well the body is managing. It might prompt you to change your diet or modify your drinking habits. It may even help you to spot an early symptom of a more serious medical condition which you can then discuss with your doctor. It's a quick, free and easy home test to perform and you'll be amazed at the insight it can give you.

Urine

Traditionally, a urine sample was always part of a doctor's examination. Today we are more likely to use a urine analysis stick (see urine test opposite) but we can still tell a lot from the colour of urine, its smell and its clarity. Normal urine is a clear light yellow with a characteristic odour.

Colour

Dark yellow
This normally shows lack of sufficient water in your diet. Apart from drinking more of it, try cutting down on alcohol, coffee, soft drinks and tea (except most herbal teas), all of which will dehydrate you further.

Bright yellow
This is often caused by taking vitamin B or a multivitamin and shouldn't be cause for concern.

Red
Often indicates recent intake of beetroot – otherwise, it could be due to blood. This is normal for women having their period but could also be due to infection or a more serious problem. Check this with the multistix (see urine test opposite) and then see your doctor.

Smell

Strong
A strong smell can indicate that you are dehydrated, have an infection, are taking hormones, or are on a high-protein diet.

Sweet
If your urine smells sweet, this could indicate diabetes (many years ago this was one of the main methods of diagnosis for the disease). You can check this with a multistix but then see your doctor.

Doctors use multistix, which display a variety of colours according to the condition being treated. You can now test yourself at home using these – the kits are stocked by most chemists.

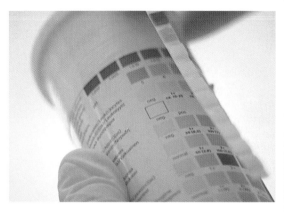

Apart from testing urine for blood, glucose and a whole range of infections, this method also tests for acidity, dehydration, bilirubin (a sign of possible liver disease) and protein (which may indicate kidney problems). In all cases, you may well have a handy indication of any problem, but testing should always be followed up by a visit to your doctor for confirmation. While many disorders that show up in the urine are minor and easily treatable, others are potentially serious.

Clarity

Cloudy urine usually denotes an infection or protein in the urine. To differentiate between the two, test with the multistix (see above). If it is caused by an infection then you will test positive for leucocytes and/or blood and protein. If leucocytes aren't present, but it is positive for protein, then you may have a problem with your kidneys. In either case you should see your doctor to be checked.

If you do have an infection then you should avoid coffee and orange juice and replace with cranberry juice (sugar-free preferably) and drink up to one litre per day. Taking vitamin C acidifies the urine and can be helpful. If you choose to take antibiotics either from your doctor or from over the counter in the chemist, make sure you follow that with eating natural yoghurt (without the fruit or sugar) and/or acidophilus supplements to replace good bowel bacteria.

If you would prefer not to take antibiotics then take uva ursi (a herb that is powerful against urinary infections) or echinacea for a week. If your symptoms worsen, or are not better within a week, see your doctor. Always see the doctor if you are pregnant or have a fever with cloudy urine.

Cloudy urine in women can also be associated with menstruation or a yeast infection in the vagina. If it is a yeast infection you will probably also have a white discharge and itching. Vaginal yeast infections always come from the gut so you need to change your diet as well as take local preparations, such as Diflucan or Canesten, which your chemist can supply. Cut out sugar, bread, wine and beer from your diet for two weeks, eat natural yoghurt (sugar-free) and take acidophilus daily to replace good bowel bacteria.

urine

Bowel movements

Just looking at your bowel movements can give you a lot of information about your digestive system. The characteristics to look for are colour, consistency, volume, presence of blood and mucus on the outside of the stool, presence of undigested food (surprisingly common), and smell.

Colour

Stools should be a dark brown.

Red streaks

These could indicate a large intake of red-coloured food, such as beetroots or tomatoes; or blood from the colon – which may signify a benign condition like haemorrhoids or a polyp, or something more serious.

Black

A black stool could indicate a large intake of dark-coloured foods such as liquorice or blueberries; iron supplements or bismuth containing antacids; or blood from higher in the gastro-intestinal (GI) tract, which could be caused by a bleeding stomach or duodenal ulcer.

Pale or clay-coloured

This may indicate an inability to absorb fats properly, an intake of antacids containing aluminium hydroxide, the result of a recent barium test in the GI tract, certain weight loss medication, liver disease, or coeliac disease (related to gluten intolerance).

Green

A green stool is very common in breast-fed infants but rare in adults. It may indicate an infection, a rapid transit time (see page 65), or a large intake of green leafy vegetables.

Consistency

Believe it or not, there is a standard scale for stool consistency, the Bristol Stool Scales (opposite top), which indicates digestion time for food. Type 1 has been digested the longest, type 7 the shortest. The ideal is type 3 or 4.

Whether stools are formed or loose depends to a large extent on your diet and the state of your friendly bowel bacteria. If you are on a high-protein, high-dairy diet, you are more likely to have a formed stool. On the other hand, if you are a vegetarian, it is likely to be looser.

If you have food intolerances or a poor digestion, you are likely to have an intermittently loose stool. If you don't drink much plain water and drink a lot of alcohol, coffee, tea etc, then your stool is likely to lack fluid, be drier, and therefore more formed.

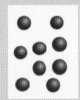

Type 1

Separate hard lumps, like nuts

Type 2

Sausage-like but lumpy

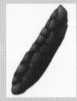

Type 3

Like a sausage but with cracks in the surface

Type 4

Like a snake or sausage, smooth and soft

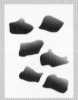

Type 5

Soft blobs with clear-cut edges

Type 6

Fluffy pieces with ragged edges, a mushy stool

Type 7

Watery, no solid pieces

Volume

The average volume of stool passed is 100g (3½ oz) – the size of a big sausage. Extra volume may indicate an infection. If the stool changes from dry and hard to a more normal consistency, this can indicate that your diet has improved, since normal stools will be larger in volume than a constipated stool, which lacks water and fibre.

Blood and/or mucus on the outside of the stool

If the blood is fresh, then it is usually from a fissure or haemorrhoid in the anus or a tiny tear in the anal canal from a hard stool. It can also be due to a more serious disease. Mucus is always produced by the body to remove threatening toxins such as bacteria, viruses or irritants. On the outside of the stool it can be associated with active inflammatory bowel disease or parasites. It can also be seen with infections. If either blood or mucus persists, you should consult your doctor.

Presence of undigested food

Often you will see nuts, seeds, pieces of corn or tomato – all these signify that you are not digesting your food as well as you should. It is usually associated with not chewing your food well, poor stomach acid and/or lack of digestive enzymes.

Smell

Stools are never exactly fragrant, but their smell can become exceptionally unpleasant. This is usually due to poor digestion, constipation, altered bowel flora, or toxicity in the bowel due to poor bowel health.

The section on digestion (pages 64–87) has action plans to remedy many of the conditions mentioned here. However, if your stool suggests something more serious, consult your doctor.

bowel movements

Bad breath

Another thing the body expels is of course breath – and bad breath is a problem for many people. Very often they are unaware of it until someone else points it out. Like body odour, most people approach it by buying something to take the odour away but in fact it often reflects an internal problem.

The most common causes for bad breath are in or around the mouth: gum disease, mouth infection, nose or throat infection, poor oral hygiene, tooth decay, tooth abscess or catarrh.

Less commonly known causes arise in the digestive system: excess sugar in the diet, parasites in the digestive tract, overgrowth of abnormal bacteria in the gut, low stomach acid leading to poor digestion of protein, low digestive enzymes and liver or kidney disease.

 ## Fresh breath action plan

+ Visit your dentist and dental hygienist regularly.

+ Brush your teeth, at least twice a day, preferably after every meal.

+ Replace your tooth brush every 3 months.

+ Floss your teeth daily particularly after meals when food can get stuck in your teeth.

+ Avoid spicy, strong-flavoured foods such as anchovies, blue cheese, salami and garlic. These can leave odours in your mouth that linger for hours.

+ Avoid foods (mainly high sugar) that promote tooth decay.

+ Chew your food thoroughly to help digestion.

+ Take a digestive enzyme to improve digestion if chewing isn't enough.

+ Take acidophilus to help create good bowel bacteria.

+ Take more vitamin C by eating more vegetables and fruit and by taking supplements if you have an active mouth infection.

If these tips aren't enough, then visit your dentist first and then your doctor.

Bad breath often reflects an internal problem

✚ Testing your mineral levels

Along with the tongue and breath, our taste can also provide an indication of what is going on within our bodies. Our bodies have an innate wisdom within them which registers what we need at any time. Our taste buds on our tongues and surrounding tissues in the mouth help us to register these bodily needs. This then encourages us to go and get the food we need.

One of the things that many people are deficient in these days is minerals. Yet minerals are essential for life in all plants and animals. Considering how essential they are, how have we become deficient in them? Unfortunately modern farming is partly to blame, as this has increasingly depleted the soil of vital minerals, while many people's lifestyles and food choices tend to rob the body of minerals (and vitamins too).

Some people believe that if you lose just one of the trace minerals then metabolic performance declines by 50 per cent. It will also make you crave food, causing you to overeat – which is why getting your mineral levels balanced is very important. Certainly, most people have more energy and enjoyment of life when they are not mineral deficient. Regular testing can be very useful as most people have an imbalance in one or more of their minerals unless they are taking steps to replace them.

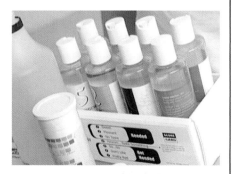

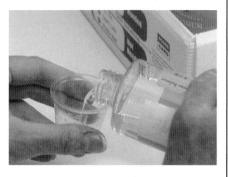

To do this test you need to order the mineral taste testing kit (see page 218). In this kit you will get eight different bottles of minerals. To test, you put a small amount from each bottle in a glass and then drink it. Do not take something else at the time. Then record the taste. The sweeter the taste the more you need it, the more foul tasting the less you need it, but, to be sure, look at the chart enclosed with the kit.

Then eat a diet rich in the foods that you need and also take supplements. Retest weekly until you are back to normal.

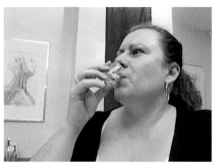

How yo
body w

Your body is a fantastic piece of work – your heart beats, your blood goes around, your lungs breathe, and your digestion gurgles away. Most of the time we don't have to think about all those bodily functions but there comes a time when what we do and what we eat finally shows up in the body: it's put on a lot weight, the stomach is griping, joints are creaking, and you feel older than your years, worn-out and low-spirited. But it doesn't have to be like this. Once you understand how your body works, you'll know how diet and exercise really affect it, and you'll be able to take control of your own health and wellbeing – for the rest of your life.

ur
orks

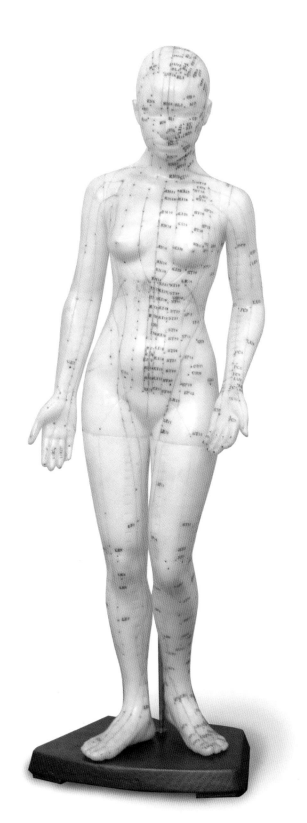

Heart and circulation
Your lifeblood

This is the beating heart of us – pumping blood through a network of veins, arteries and capillaries, carrying nourishment to every part of our body. It's literally our lifeblood but too many of us take it for granted. In the western world more people die of heart attacks, strokes and bloodvessel diseases than any other condition. Get to know what you should and shouldn't do for a healthy heart and circulation, and follow the Cardio-vascular action plan to stave off everything from heart attacks to varicose veins.

Heart of gold

The heart is an everlasting symbol of romance and true love – and a highly efficient fuel pump. The heart keeps the rest of the body going. About the size of a closed fist, it's made mostly of muscle fibres, which can contract continuously, regularly and rhythmically at an average rate of 70 to 80 beats per minute, for a lifetime. It's divided into four chambers – two pairs either side of a vertical muscular wall. The upper pair, the left and right atrium, are the receiving chambers for blood, while the lower pair, the left and right ventricle, are the pumping chambers. A number of valves ensure that the blood flows in only one direction.

The left side of the heart is more powerful than the right, and pumps blood that has been oxygenated by the lungs to the whole body, via the aorta (the main blood vessel). The right side sends blood via the pulmonary artery to the lungs, where it is oxygenated and then sent to the left side of the heart.

At rest, the heart moves about 70ml of blood (half a teacupful) per contraction and five litres of blood per minute. The body's total blood volume is 5 litres, so effectively the heart pumps the entire body's blood volume in one minute: this figure is known as the cardiac output. During exercise this figure may rise to 25 to 30 litres of blood per minute, depending on the level of fitness. As you get fitter, the heart's left ventricle will enlarge and so pump out more blood on each contraction. This allows the heart rate per minute to drop, which consumes less energy. In fact, the cardiac output during exercise for an athlete may be double that of a sedentary person, and this will be achieved mainly by enlargement of the left ventricle.

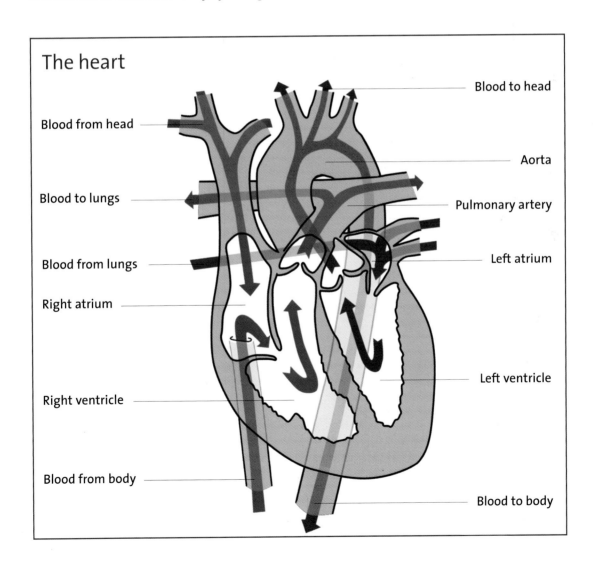

The heart

Blood from head

Blood to lungs

Blood from lungs

Right atrium

Right ventricle

Blood from body

Blood to head

Aorta

Pulmonary artery

Left atrium

Left ventricle

Blood to body

This powerful pump, which never switches off, consumes a lot of fuel itself, so requires its own blood supply. This is provided by two coronary arteries, the left and the right, the left being the more important, carrying 60 to 70 per cent of the blood. It's these arteries that tend to get blocked, so we need to look after them.

A web of blood

Arteries run parallel with veins throughout the body – they're connected by capillaries in a huge, complex network. After the exchange of oxygen and carbon dioxide has taken place, veins transport the deoxygenated blood back to the heart. A system of valves ensures that this waste-rich blood always flows in the right direction, and also supports the blood in moving against gravity. As the walls of the veins are fairly thin, and blood is a dark maroon colour, the veins under the skin show up quite clearly.

Capillaries are thinner yet – much thinner than arteries and veins and very fragile – in fact, they are barely one cell thick, which means that blood cells can pass through them only in single file. Their thin walls allow the exchange of oxygen and carbon dioxide: the oxygen-rich red blood cells from the artery release their oxygen into the surrounding tissue. The tissue on the other hand releases its waste products such as carbon dioxide, and this is then taken up by the red blood cells in the vein.

Cardiovascular disease

In the western world, cardiovascular disease is still the number one killer. In Britain alone there are about 268,000 heart attacks each year, of which around 147,000 are in men and 121,000 in women, while many more people live daily with angina. Like heart attacks, strokes don't always kill but they are the leading cause of chronic severe disability in Britain.

The chief cause of cardiovascular disease is atherosclerosis, commonly known as 'furring of the arteries', which affects almost all of us and is increasingly being seen in childhood. It is generally progressive with age and there may be a strong family predisposition.

This 'furring' is the build-up of plaque in the medium and large arteries, which slows down the normal flow of blood. The plaque, which is made up of cholesterol, calcium and platelets, may grow slowly over the years and create a gradual blockage, until there is a severe narrowing or total blockage; or it may become more calcified, breaking off a piece that travels downstream and causes a heart attack or stroke by blocking the relevant arteries. Either way, its progress is normally unnoticeable until the blood supply to an affected part is severely impeded.

Although many arteries can be affected, plaque is most dangerous in the coronary arteries and the neck arteries (vertebral and carotid) or their branches. Atherosclerosis of these two systems is what contributes to angina, heart attacks and strokes.

✚ Taking the pulse

When you take your pulse, you're measuring the contractions in the artery wall that occur each time the heart beats. This is how it works:

The heart pumps blood out to the body via the aorta or main artery, which branches into smaller arteries which reach the whole body. Arteries have three layers, including an elastic and very strong middle muscular layer which helps the heart pump the blood. When the heart beats, this layer relaxes to accommodate the blood, and then contracts once the heart relaxes to move the blood along. It is these contractions, which mirror the heartbeats, that you're feeling when you take your pulse.

Angina

If you get a severe pain in the centre of your chest when you're exercising or stressed, then you may be suffering with angina.

Angina occurs when a coronary artery is partially blocked, causing reduced oxygen flow to the heart muscle cells, which are then weakened but not killed. This severe pain, which often feels like a vice, may be felt in the left arm, jaw or neck. Although it is typically triggered by exercise and stress, it can be brought on more quickly by cold weather and by exercise after a heavy meal. For the latter reason it can sometimes be mistaken for heartburn, which also gives you a severe pain in the centre of your chest (see page 76). If your pain stops when you rest, then it is more likely to be angina, and if it stops when you take an antacid, then it is more likely to be indigestion.

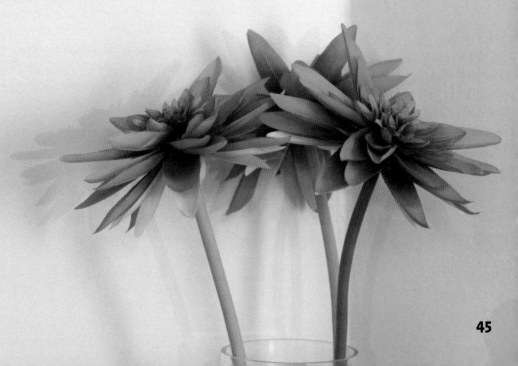

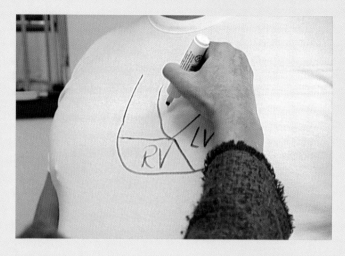

Dr Wendy sketches out the location and size of his heart for Daniel Davis

Heart attacks

Most people know when they are having a heart attack. They get a severe pain in the centre of the chest, like angina, but usually more severe, which lasts for longer than half an hour and may be accompanied by sweating, nausea, dizziness and pain down the left arm. This is caused by a complete blockage in a coronary artery, which kills the heart muscle (this is myocardial infarction). The left coronary artery and its branches, taking the greater part of the blood, get blocked more often. (Many people think that when they have a heart attack that the aorta or pulmonary artery gets blocked, but in fact it is the coronary arteries, which are much smaller.)

What happens after a heart attack depends on which part of the heart is involved, but many deaths are due to the effect on the conduction system, leading to irregular pumping of the heart.

Keeping the beat

The heart's beating is controlled by a specialised conduction system, centred in the right atrium, which normally makes all four chambers of the heart beat together. The average resting heart rate is between 60 and 80 beats per minute (sometimes lower in athletes) but rises with exercise and emotion, when hormones such as adrenaline are released.

Most of us become aware of our heartbeat during activity or high emotion but if you are still conscious of your heart beating during a rest period and your pulse is faster than 100 beats per minute then you may be suffering with palpitations. These can be caused by a rapid heartbeat, irregular heartbeat or extra heartbeat. If you have this you should see your doctor as prolonged or persistent palpitations can be caused by thyroid disease, heart valve disease or a conduction problem.

The thing to remember about palpitations is that they're usually made worse by stress, coffee, alcohol even in moderate amounts, B vitamin deficiencies and low levels of magnesium and potassium.

Palpitations action plan

+ Take more B vitamins – commonly depleted by a vegetarian diet and alcohol consumption – found in wholegrains and meat.

+ Take more magnesium – found in nuts, seeds and green leafy vegetables.

+ Take more potassium – found in bananas, watercress and courgettes.

Strokes

Strokes are the third most common cause of death in the western world, after heart disease and cancer. They are, however, the commonest cause of severe chronic disability, affecting two in every 1,000 people. They are twice as common in black people than in white, and 75 per cent of sufferers are over 65 years old.

They occur when a part of the brain is deprived of oxygen and essential nutrients, due to a blood vessel in the brain being blocked, or because of damage to the brain from a haemorrhage. Cerebral haemorrhage, or bleeding into the brain, is usually the most serious kind of stroke and is often fatal. It is commonly the result of a small artery rupturing, having been previously weakened by atherosclerosis, and then further stressed by high blood pressure.

Much more common than a cerebral haemorrhage is a blockage of one of the brain arteries, arising from either plaque or a brain clot. This may occur in people with atherosclerosis of the carotid or vertebral arteries or one of their branches. It may also be caused by a brain clot being sent up to the brain from the heart, from diseased heart valves or irregular heart rates.

As atherosclerosis is the most common predisposing factor to these serious cardiovascular diseases, how do you avoid getting it in the first place? The following risk factors include the usual suspects:

+ Smoking

+ High blood pressure

+ Diabetes

+ Obesity

+ Stress

+ Lack of exercise

+ Diet high in saturated fats

+ High levels of cholesterol, homocysteine or C reactive protein (see overleaf)

How important is cholesterol?

It's true that raised cholesterol is an important risk factor for heart disease, but half the people who die of a heart attack will have had normal cholesterol. Cholesterol is vital in many ways: it's used in cell membranes, the formation of certain hormones and the protective coverings of nerves, and it's required in the production of vitamin D.

About 80 per cent of total body cholesterol is manufactured in the liver, while 20 per cent comes from the diet. This is why diet has some effect on lowering levels – decreasing your intake of animal protein, alcohol and sugar certainly helps – but other factors, such as family history and exercise, are involved.

Crucially there are two main types of cholesterol, and you need to distinguish between them, LDLs (low density lipoproteins) are 'bad' cholesterol and HDLs (high density lipoproteins) are 'good' cholesterol. LDLs take cholesterol from the liver to all cells of the body to make cell membranes, vitamin D, hormones and nerve coverings. HDLs carry any cholesterol that hasn't been used by the cells on to the liver to be recycled. Normally this system is in balance but if there are not enough HDLs to mop up the extra cholesterol then the cholesterol will form plaque that will stick to the artery walls.

For this reason, as several studies have proved, the most important risk factor for cardiovascular disease in women is their HDL cholesterol level, and their HDL/total cholesterol ratio. This appears to be more important than their overall levels of cholesterol – an important fact to grasp in this day and age when anyone can buy cholesterol-lowering drugs over the counter.

But concentration on cholesterol may have diverted attention from other important causes of cardiovascular disease, not as well known to most people: high blood homocysteine and high blood C reactive protein.

Homocysteine

High levels of homocysteine, an amino acid, in the blood can raise the risk of heart disease and stroke as much as smoking a pack of cigarettes per day, having a high blood pressure of 160/95 and having a very raised cholesterol level. In fact, it may be a bigger risk factor than raised cholesterol. About 10 per cent of the population have high levels of homocysteine. There's a strong genetic influence although lifestyle factors are, as ever, important. A diet high in animal proteins, smoking and lack of exercise also contribute, as well as medication such as steroids, methotrexate, phenytoin and tricyclic antidepressants.

Homocysteine is made in the body from methionine, which is found in large supplies in meat, cheese, dairy and eggs. Your body naturally converts it into glutathione, the most important antioxidant, and SAMe, a vital brain and body chemical acting as an antidepressant and anti-arthritic. The problems arise when it is not converted properly (for this you need to have

✚ Homeocysteine test

This test is relatively new in Britain although other countries have used it for a long time. It involves taking a pinprick sample of blood from a finger, and applying it to a spot on a card. This is then sent off to the laboratory (see page 218) with a request form, and within two weeks you will receive a result telling you what your level is.
Note: This test is only a rough guide as homocysteine can be more accurately measured by sending a blood sample directly to the lab, as your doctor would do.

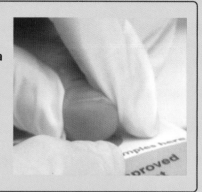

adequate levels of B vitamins and zinc). The homocysteine that accumulates in the body can do all kinds of damage, including: injuring and irritating the arteries; contributing to the build-up of plaque in the arteries; causing the blood to thicken and stick to the arterial wall; oxidising cholesterol, which makes it more dangerous; promoting inflammation in the body which, in the long run, can damage joints, arteries and nerves; and increasing the risk of Alzheimer's disease and declining memory.

To reduce homocysteine, follow the general Cardiovascular action plan on page 54, and try the following supplements:

- ✚ Folic acid
- ✚ Vitamin B complex
- ✚ Zinc picolinate or food state zinc

C reactive protein

C reactive protein (CRP) is an inflammatory marker found in the blood. It is raised in any situation where there is inflammation in the body, such as an acute viral attack, or in chronic situations such as rheumatoid arthritis and gout. In some, particularly obese people, the inflammatory markers will be elevated even without a distinct disease diagnosis being made. CRP, except in the acute situation, is now being recognised as an important independent predictor of cardiovascular death risk.

If your level is above 5mg/l, then you are four times more likely to die from a cardiovascular cause.

Guard against this by following the Cardiovascular action plan on page 50, and specifically take omega-3 essential fatty acids. For further suggestions see the anti-inflammatory diet, page 123.

Cardiovascular action plan

Lowering your risk of heart disease requires a comprehensive approach:

+ Stop smoking.

+ Reduce consumption of animal products.

+ Reduce alcohol, which depletes the body of B vitamins, zinc and magnesium.

+ Eliminate sugar.

+ Eat at least 6 to 8 helpings of fruit and vegetables per day.

+ Increase fibre in diet to eliminate excess cholesterol from the diet.

+ Reduce caffeine to lower homocysteine and CRP.

+ Eliminate soft caffeinated drinks.

+ Eliminate any food high in saturated fats, particularly deep-fried food.

+ Keep your weight within a BMI of 25 (see page 14).

+ Reduce stress by making time for yoga, massage or tai chi.

+ Exercise regularly.

+ If you have diabetes, keep it under tight control (see page 100).

+ Get your blood pressure checked regularly, and keep it below 140/80 (see page 52).

Supplements for the heart

+ A good multimineral and vitamin to replace any deficiencies
+ Vitamin E to improve circulation
+ Magnesium for blood pressure and stress reduction
+ B vitamins, particularly if homocysteine is high
+ Coenzyme Q10 – aids heart function and lowers blood pressure
+ Fish oils for good circulation

80 per cent of people with high blood pressure can be treated by a significant change in lifestyle

High blood pressure

Everyone knows they should get their blood pressure checked, but how many people actually do it? And why it is so important?

It's having high blood pressure that rings warning bells (low blood pressure doesn't have the same health implications). Sustained high blood pressure damages the blood vessels, promoting hardening of the arteries. This makes it a major risk factor for a heart attack and stroke. Indeed, it is the most important risk factor for stroke, making you seven times more likely to suffer one. High blood pressure can also severely damage the heart, kidneys and eyes. And all the while you may never know what's happening. You may notice a headache, nosebleed, dizziness or sweating as a result of high blood pressure, but most people experience no symptoms at all. This is why it is important to get it checked regularly.

The blood pressure check is essentially a measurement of how much pressure it takes to stop the flow of blood through the arteries, and therefore how much loss of flexibility there is in the system. There are two measurements: the systolic or top figure, which is taken at the moment when the heart beats, when the pressure is at its highest; and the diastolic, at the time the heart is at rest between beats, when the blood pressure is at its lowest. The results are given as the systolic reading 'over' the diastolic reading – like this: 140/80.

Blood pressure goes up slowly and steadily as we age, but it also fluctuates on a day-to-day, minute-to-minute basis. Your blood pressure is usually at its lowest when you first get up in the morning and tends to get higher as the day progresses. It is also affected by anxiety, stress and activity. As blood pressure varies so much during the day, it is important to get several readings in different settings before diagnosing blood pressure problems. For this reason – and because some people's blood pressure goes up when they go to the doctor's (so-called 'white-coat blood pressure') – home monitoring can be very useful.

While genetics and lifestyle factors account for most incidences of high blood pressure, about 10 per cent are due to an underlying medical condition of the kidneys, thyroid or adrenal glands, which must be treated professionally. High blood pressure can also be a side effect of medication such as the birth control pill, hormone replacement therapy and some antidepressants; again, regular checking is essential.

Eighty per cent of people with high blood pressure fall into the category of mild to moderate, with measurements being lower than 180/115. Most of these people can be treated as effectively by a significant change in lifestyle as by taking drugs. There have been a number of studies showing how following the right eating plan for lowering your blood pressure can stop and possibly even reverse hardening of the arteries.

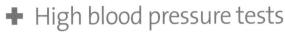

✚ High blood pressure tests

Check your pulse – do this when you're rested, and haven't eaten, drunk, smoked or exercised for the last half hour. A normal pulse should be between 60 and 80 beats per minute. If your pulse is consistently above 80 or irregular, you should check your blood pressure and consult your doctor. Most chemists stock a range of blood pressure monitors that you can use at home – go for one that measures pressure at the upper arm rather than the wrist. As with taking your pulse, don't eat, drink, smoke or exercise for half an hour before taking your blood pressure. Also, check your magnesium levels (see page 39), as this mineral is very important in helping to keep your pulse steady and your blood pressure down.

Adult blood pressure measurements:

Normal	about 120/80, to upper limit of 140/90
Borderline high	140/95 to 160/95
Moderately high	160/95 to 180/115
Severely high	over 180/115

You can make a difference by following the Cardiovascular action plan. Make a point of eating more oily fish and lots of magnesium-rich food such as whole grains, nuts, and green leafy vegetables. Apples are also good as they contain pectin which helps reduce blood pressure. It helps to have a salt-free diet – so absolutely no fast food, convenience food, junk foods, diet drinks and the MSG you get in Chinese takeaways. Finally, avoid medications that put up your blood pressure, e.g. antihistamines, ibuprofen and the other nonsteroidal anti-inflammatories.

If you're taking diuretics, then make sure you have your potassium and magnesium levels checked. Diuretics can lower levels of these important minerals, precipitating heart palpitations or irregular rhythms.

If you snore heavily, you should get your blood pressure checked – heavy snorers are more likely to have high blood pressure and angina. See also the section on sleep apnoea (page 113) to see if you may have this problem. If you suspect you do, discuss with your doctor, as blood pressure often returns to normal if you treat the sleep disorder.

Supplements for high blood pressure

- ✚ Magnesium
- ✚ Fish oil or flaxseed oil
- ✚ Coenzyme supplement, especially for those taking a statin cholesterol-lowering drug (40 per cent of people with high blood pressure have a low level)

Varicose veins

While atherosclerotic damage to blood vessels can go unnoticed, varicose veins are all too evident – those rather unsightly bulging veins in the lower legs. They occur in many women, particularly over the age of 35 and after multiple pregnancies, and affect 60 per cent of adults in Britain. Varicose veins are often accompanied by dull, nagging aches and pains and a sensation of heaviness in the legs. If they get very severe they can produce ankle swelling, leg sores or ulcers.

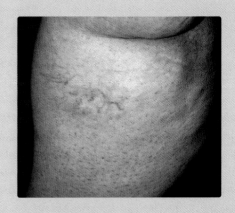

Varicose veins are produced when the vein wall is weakened, and so the valves in the veins, which are returning the blood to the heart from the tissues, stretch and can't close properly. This then allows blood to accumulate in the veins, causing enlargement.

While genes are a factor, as well as pregnancy, varicose veins are also common in obese people, due to their extra weight, along with people who are constipated or eat a poor diet. This is particularly true if the diet is lacking in vitamin C and bioflavonoid (found in citrus fruits and dark red berries), as these strengthen the collagen structure in the vein walls. Poor circulation is another major factor, and so they are more common in people who sit cross-legged, or stand in one position for prolonged periods. If you have to stand all day, consider wearing support stockings (never tight pop socks). Avoid heavy lifting and, after a hot bath or shower, douse your legs in cold water for two minutes as this improves the circulation. For all-round improvement, follow the Cardiovascular and Constipation action plans on pages 48 and 71.

 ## Supplements for varicose veins

+ Vitamin E to help circulation and to make collagen

+ Rutin, a potent bioflavonoid

+ Coenzyme Q10 to improve tissue oxygenation and circulation

+ Horse chestnut seeds to help seal the leaky veins and capillaries, protect the vein walls against damage, and reduce swelling

If your condition doesn't improve, then consider seeing your doctor to discuss other treatments. In general, varicose veins are a cosmetic matter and don't pose a serious health problem. Obese people, however, may develop deep vein clots, ulcers and dermatitis in the ankle region.

If varicose veins do become a problem, some simple remedies may help. Avoid scratching the skin above the veins as this can cause ulceration and bleeding. To soothe inflamed veins, gently rub them with a cloth dipped in a mixture of half a teaspoonful of horse chestnut powder and two cups of water.

Respiration
A breath of fresh air

Breathing is so vital to life that it's a good job we don't have to think about it all the time – our body does it automatically. But sometimes the system we take for granted goes wrong. Have you ever had an asthma attack, when you just couldn't get enough air into your lungs? Or has something sparked off a panic attack, making you breathe so quickly and deeply that you felt dizzy and faint? At such times your respiratory system is under great stress, and it helps to know how to get it back to normal. Your lungs have enough to handle anyway – what with dust, bacteria, smoke and other toxins in the atmosphere – so learn what they love and you'll live better and breathe easy.

The lungs

Oxygen is one thing that can't be stored in the body for longer than a few minutes. That's why we have to keep breathing it in, to provide all our cells and organs with the fuel they need to stay alive. At the same time, we have to get rid of the carbon dioxide and other toxic waste that's built up in the body, so we breathe it out. A vital double balancing act for the lungs.

The oxygen-rich air we breathe in reaches the lungs via the trachea (windpipe), which runs from the neck into the chest. Further down, the trachea divides into the left and right bronchi (air passages), which enter the

The lungs

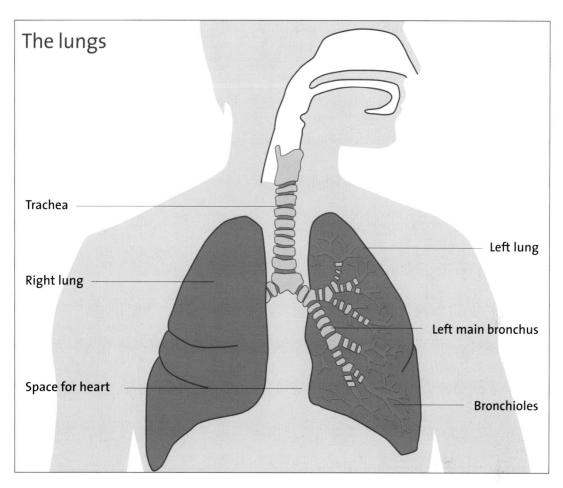

Trachea

Right lung

Space for heart

Left lung

Left main bronchus

Bronchioles

right and left lungs respectively. The bronchi then branch into smaller and smaller bronchi which then branch into bronchioles. The bronchioles finally end in tiny air sacs called alveoli where the exchange of oxygen and carbon dioxide takes place.

Each lung has about 400 to 600 million alveoli which, if laid out flat, would cover a tennis court. Oxygen passes through the wall of each alveolus into the tiny capillaries that surround it. The oxygen enters the blood in the tiny capillaries, combining with the red blood cells to travel around the body. At the same time the carbon dioxide is unloaded from the blood into the alveoli to be breathed out. These capillaries are so small that, amazingly, the blood cells have to travel through in single file.

As a result of their role in removing carbon dioxide, the lungs also have a crucial part in regulating the body's pH – its balance of acid and alkaline. Our breathing is controlled by the respiratory centre in the brain which sends signals to the body to adjust the rate of breathing to provide enough oxygen for all our different activities. When we exercise we breathe faster and more deeply to bring in more oxygen and expel more carbon dioxide. Sometimes, though, the breathing regulator goes haywire.

respiration

When stress makes you hyperventilate, grab a paper bag

Hyperventilation

If you become highly emotionally stressed or very anxious, you may start to hyperventilate, that is taking quick, deep breaths from the top of your chest. This lowers the level of carbon dioxide in the blood which causes the arteries to constrict, slowing the flow of blood through the body. This then limits how much oxygen gets to the brain and body, causing in the first instance faintness, dizziness, pressure across the chest and a feeling of shortness of breath. Later it may include tingling in the hands. This can make you feel even more panicky.

When you're in this state, you have to control your breathing, and there's a simple procedure for this. You just need to breathe into a paper bag, scrunching the opening round your mouth and nose to stop the air escaping. As you breathe in and out, you'll be inhaling into your lungs exhaled air that is rich in carbon dioxide. This will increase carbon dioxide in the blood, which signals the brain to slow your breathing – so shortening what can be a very distressing experience.

It's also possible to breathe out too little carbon dioxide rather than too much, and this is usually combined with breathing in too little oxygen. There are a number of conditions that cause this, most commonly obesity and asthma.

 How to breathe

Most people breathe incorrectly either due to chronic stress and hyperventilation or through habit.

+ The diaphragm is critical to breathing. It works together with the rib muscles to allow the chest cavity to expand with inhalation and contract with exhalation.

+ The correct way to breathe is to **blow the stomach out** during inhalation, this allows the dome of the diaphragm to flatten completely and the rib cage to expand. This allows maximum air to be brought into the lungs. On exhalation, **the stomach is pulled in**, which raises the diaphragm and returns the rib cage to its original position.

+ To learn how to breathe correctly you could attend a yoga class or see a yoga practitioner.

✚ Lung function tests

If you suspect you have asthma, then you should discuss your symptoms with your doctor, who will listen to your chest, take your peak flow and may prescribe inhalers to treat the condition. Following the lung health action plan will also be very helpful. You can keep tabs on your condition at home by doing your own peak flow testing, which measures how much air you can exhale in one breath and can be used by anyone wanting to test their lung function.

Most chemists stock peak flow machines, which cost about £12. To do the test, take a deep breath in and then breathe out as hard as you can into a mouthpiece. On the side of the machine is a scale where you can see your reading. It's usually recommended that you take the best of three readings.

Another way of testing how well your lungs work is the step test, which shows how quickly you get out of breath when you're exerting yourself (see page 192). Make a record of your time then, as you follow the exercise and eating programmes recommended in this book and get fitter and lose weight, measure your time again, and see if it's changed – it should have!

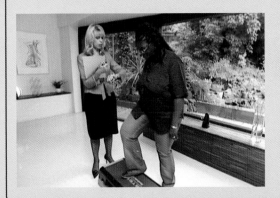 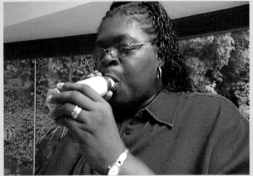

Problems for the overweight

When you're overweight or obese, there are a number of changes in the lungs that make breathing difficult. Fat accumulates in the chest wall and the abdomen, making it difficult for the chest to expand as much as it should (this is called chest splinting). The lungs are then unable to exchange air efficiently, which means that less oxygen is taken into the blood and less carbon dioxide excreted. This leads to shortness of breath or fatigue after minimal effort. It can also cause daytime sleepiness and depression, not to mention more rapid aging.

respiration

Asthma

Being overweight also increases your chance of getting asthma, the chronic respiratory condition that causes shortage of breath, wheezing, coughing and a feeling of never being able to empty the lungs. Asthma is caused by a release of inflammatory chemicals in the lungs, which then leads to varying degrees of constriction of the bronchi. Overweight people have an increased amount of inflammatory chemicals in their body, which naturally makes them more susceptible to asthma. Another exacerbating factor is their poor breathing caused by chest splinting.

The risk of asthma rises even more if you're not only overweight but also female. The reason for this is not entirely clear, but it is associated with a change in airways constriction and hormones. If you already have asthma then being overweight makes it worse.

The incidence of asthma in all groups of people has increased exponentially over the last ten years and nobody knows exactly why. In the UK it affects 4.6 million people. Attacks can be set off by a variety of triggers, such as:

+ Allergic reactions (commonly to animal fur, dust mites and food)
+ Stress
+ Chemicals and pollution
+ Respiratory infections
+ Exercise

Certainly, air pollution plays a big part with asthma – just imagine what else enters your lungs with oxygen. With each breath comes a cocktail of dust, bacteria, viruses, pollens, smoke, lead, toxic chemicals and a host of other nasty substances. So not only do the lungs supply oxygen and remove waste and poisons from the body, they also have to defend it against hostile intruders. To this end, the respiratory tract is lined with tiny hairs, called cilia, which trap foreign particles on their way to the lungs. If you smoke, these protective cilia are flattened – after you give up, they take about three months to regain their function.

Supplements for asthma

To support the immune system:

+ A high-dose multivitamin and mineral
+ Vitamin C

To inhibit the inflammatory chemicals:

+ Fish oils
+ Bromelain
+ Quercetin

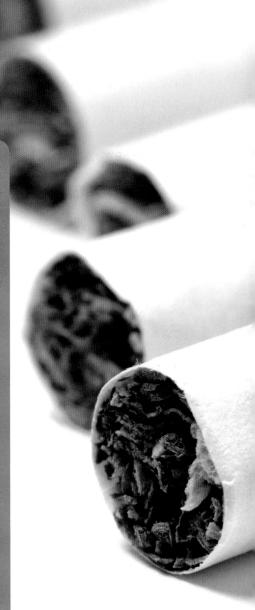

Asthma action plan

- + Don't smoke and avoid second-hand smoke.

- + Expose yourself to clean and fresh air as much as possible.

- + Protect your lungs when exposed to polluted air or toxic chemicals by wearing a properly fitting protective mask over your mouth and nose.

- + Keep an eye on your weight, particularly the size of your stomach.

- + Remove dairy foods from the diet, particularly cheese, as they tend to produce mucus that thickens secretions in the bronchi.

- + Look for and treat any food allergies.

- + Keep your salt intake low as salt makes you oversensitive to inflammatory chemicals.

- + Reduce stress and practise relaxation.

- + Take regular exercise.

- + Keep the home dust-free – don't use down or goose-feather pillows or duvets, and think about removing carpets (which trap a lot of dust).

- + Consider acupuncture, which can be very effective.

- + Follow an anti-inflammatory diet – see page 123.

Digestion
Chew this over

What goes in must come out – simple? No. It's actually a highly complex process that can be hard to digest, in more ways than one. And for you to be healthy, it has to work properly. You can't feel at your best if you are suffering from heartburn, constipation or a sluggish liver. All the pleasure in eating and drinking is wiped out and your vitality suffers. So it pays to know just what happens to each mouthful as it passes through the digestive tract so that you can maximise what you are getting from your food.

Your digestive system

This starts working before you take a bite – with the very first thought or smell of food, which stimulates the salivary glands into action. Saliva contains digestive enzymes that start the process of digestion, particularly of carbohydrates. In order for the saliva to work, it has to mix well with the food, so thorough chewing is essential.

This may seem obvious, but in fact most of us are appalling chewers – chomping our food one, two, three times and gulping it down, expecting our stomach and intestines to do all the work. This leads to most of us eating more than we should. If we actually stopped to chew our food well, we would be more attuned to the stomach's signal that it had received enough food. The problem for most of us is that we don't realise we've eaten too much until it's too late. So if you have a poor digestive system, the first thing you have to do is **chew your food well**.

The food then travels down the oesophagus into the stomach, which is pivotal to the digestive system. It releases hydrochloric acid and is the most acidic environment in the body. Fortunately, it also produces its own mucus to protect itself from the acid.

The acid is primarily responsible for the digestion of proteins, but it also activates the production of digestive enzymes such as lipase, which digests fat. The acid in the stomach kills off any bacteria and parasites that may have invaded, and is the first line of defence of the immune system in the gut. Many vitamins and minerals require proper stomach acid in order to be properly absorbed, such as iron, calcium, folic acid and vitamin B12.

Too much or too little stomach acid?

It is always assumed that anyone who has indigestion or acid reflux is suffering from excess stomach acid but, in fact, the reverse is often true. As we age our stomach acid production goes down, particularly after the age of 50, by which time 75 per cent of the population will have low acid levels. Stomach acid production also relies on the mineral zinc and, as up to 50 per cent of the British population are deficient in zinc, we can begin to understand why low acid levels are so prevalent. Antacids also cause low-acid levels – in the UK we spend over a million pounds annually on antacids bought over the counter.

Stomach acid is also important in the digestion of protein and low levels will lead to indigestion of protein with its attendant problems. Although there are many symptoms associated with low stomach acid, the most important symptom to look for is that you may feel full earlier on during a meal because food will be kept longer in the stomach (due to a lack of stomach acid).

Because the stomach process is so important for digestion, a lack of stomach acid can have many adverse effects, not least the development of food allergies or intolerances. A recent study has shown that people who took antacids on a long-term basis had a 25 per cent increased chance of developing food intolerances (see page 69). Signs of low stomach acid include:

+ Bloating and burping
+ Fullness early on during meals
+ Multiple food sensitivities
+ Nausea after taking supplements

+ Weak, peeling and cracked fingernails
+ Acne
+ Iron deficiency
+ Undigested food in stool

High stomach acid

High stomach acid is most commonly seen in younger, more stressed people who drink too much coffee, tea and alchohol and eat spicy food. Anti-inflammatory drugs can give you the same problems as high stomach acid because they interfere with the stomach's own protection against excess acid levels. There is also a fairly strong genetic influence.

✚ Test for stomach acid

This simple test for low stomach acid should be used as a guide only. You need an empty stomach, so don't eat anything for at least four hours. Then mix a level tablespoon of bicarbonate of soda into a glass of water, drink this solution and wait 10 minutes. Generally speaking, bicarbonate is rapidly converted into gas by stomach acid (and incidentally it's a very good antacid). So if you start to belch or bloat quite quickly then you have adequate stomach acid (and once you start to react like this it can go on for an hour or so). On the other hand, if there's been no belching or bloating within 10 minutes then you have low stomach acid.

High stomach acid is associated with the development of ulcers in the stomach and duodenum and also a state of chronic inflammation in the stomach. Frequently these are associated with eating the wrong food or too much food. In 70 per cent of cases they are also thought to be associated with a bacteria, called H pylori, that invades the mucus lining of the wall of the stomach and so affects how the stomach protects itself from the acid. Duodenal ulcers have a strong genetic influence.

 # Stomach acid action plan

Low stomach acid:
Check your symptoms, and try testing yourself with the stomach acid test – if that is found to be low then try following this plan for the next month and see if your symptoms improve. If not then see your doctor.

✚ Chew your food well.

✚ Make sure you are not zinc deficient, and eat a zinc-rich diet as well as taking a zinc supplement.

✚ Take betaine hydrochloride before your meals to aid digestion.

High stomach acid:
✚ Stop smoking.

✚ Stop drinking coffee and decrease wine and beer intake.

✚ Stop eating red meat and spicy food.

✚ Reduce fat in your diet as it is hard to digest.

✚ Reduce stress.

If you suspect that you have developed an ulcer you should consult your doctor.

Your intestines

From the stomach, food passes first to the small intestine, where 90 per cent of digestion and absorption of nutrients occurs. Its walls are covered with tiny finger-like projections, called villi, so while the small intestine is about 6 metres (20 feet) long, the total area of absorption is much larger. It secretes its own variety of digesting substances as well as receiving digestive enzymes from the pancreas, liver and gallbladder.

The small intestine is divided up into three distinct sections: the duodenum, which is vital for digesting fat and neutralising stomach acid; the jejunum, which has the largest absorption area, particularly of protein, carbohydrate and water-soluble vitamins; and the ileum, where more fat is absorbed, as well as vitamin B12 and bile salts.

When the small intestine has done its work, the large intestine takes over. Starting at the appendix and ending at the rectum, it's about 1.5 metres (5 feet) long, much shorter than the small intestine but thicker. The main part of it is the colon, which absorbs any remaining water and electrolytes from the thick liquid delivered by the small intestine. It then serves as a holding tank for the waste material that will in due course be evacuated.

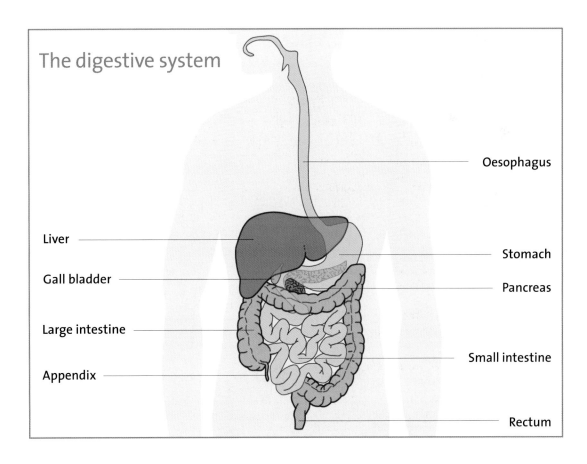

The digestive system

Oesophagus

Liver

Stomach

Gall bladder

Pancreas

Large intestine

Small intestine

Appendix

Rectum

Constipation

Opening your bowels regularly is an important factor in the maintenance of good health. In Britain, it's considered normal to have one bowel movement a day, but in fact it depends on your diet. A vegetarian diet may often lead to three to four bowel movements a day due to the high levels of fibre eaten, whereas a diet with animal protein may be more constipating. Just as important as fibre for regular bowel movements is drinking enough water and taking exercise. And magnesium plays a part too – low levels may cause constipation, so keep up your intake (see page 142).

What makes our system seize up?

Many factors have an effect on the workings of our bowels. These include:

+ Cooked cheese
+ White pasta
+ White bread and rice
+ Junk food

+ Pregnancy
+ Stress or depression
+ Thyroid disease
+ High calcium in blood

+ Iron supplements
+ Long-term use of laxatives
+ Drugs, e.g. painkillers or antidepressants

A gutful of bacteria

There's bad bacteria and there's good bacteria – and the bacteria in your gut are definitely the good guys. There are over 400 different kinds of them in your small and large intestine, many millions of each, and they play several crucial roles for us. In the small intestine they help with absorption and make critical vitamins such as the B series and vitamin K. In the large intestine they're mostly putrefying bacteria that help transform some of the toxic chemicals in the bowel. They also promote regular bowel functioning. So healthy bacteria are essential.

Opening your bowels regularly is an important factor in the maintenance of good health

14 million people in the UK suffer with constipation

Why constipation is bad for you

The waste matter held in the colon should be evacuated within 18 to 36 hours – the time it takes food to transit from one end of the digestive system to the other in the average person. After this time, harmful toxins are produced by the putrefying bacteria that work on the waste, producing foul-smelling gas. The longer the toxic material sits in your large intestine, the longer it is in contact with the lining of the gut wall, exposing it to dangerous chemicals with harmful long-term consequences, such as bowel cancer.

Another danger, for women, concerns oestrogen: if this isn't removed, it's converted by bacteria back into another form of the hormone, causing higher levels of oestrogen in the body. Breast cancer has been linked to higher levels of circulating oestrogen.

Constipation, or slow transit time, has also been linked to a wide array of conditions that may not be as serious as cancer but greatly reduce your quality of life. Symptoms include:

+ Allergies
+ Bad breath
+ Body odour
+ Depression
+ Excess gas

+ Fatigue
+ Headaches
+ High cholesterol
+ Indigestion
+ Obesity

+ Varicose veins
+ Joint pain
+ Dark circles under the eyes

+ Stool transit time

Eat some beets or corn on the cob, then watch for redness or a piece of undigested corn in your stools. You should see this being excreted within 36 hours; if not, then you have a slow transit time. Follow the guidelines for treating constipation and then repeat the test a month later. If you keep seeing redness in your stools and it's not related to eating beets, visit your doctor. See also the Bristol Stool Scales on page 37.

digestion

Constipation action plan

If you're constipated, don't automatically reach for the laxatives. People in Britain spend more money on laxatives than any other country in Europe, but as many as 80 per cent of sufferers could be cured by simple changes to diet and lifestyle.

+ Eat more fibre – 6 to 8 helpings of vegetables and fruit per day, plus wholegrains, e.g. brown rice, bran flakes and granola.

+ Drink 8 glasses of water per day.

+ Cut your caffeine intake to 2 cups of coffee or tea per day.

+ Stop drinking all soft drinks.

+ Stop eating cheese.

+ Stop eating white pasta, white rice and white bread.

+ Eat food high in pectin, e.g. apples, carrots, cabbage and okra.

+ Eat prunes, figs or raisins.

+ Walk for half an hour per day.

+ Never repress the urge to open your bowels.

 ## Supplements for constipation

If these simple measures don't work, before you reach for the laxatives try two or more of the following:

+ Aloe vera juice is a natural laxative with a healing and cleansing effect on the digestive system.

+ Acidophilus helps keep the bacteria healthy in the gut.

+ Freshly ground flaxseed or flaxseed oil helps to soften the stools.

+ Psyllium husk – take it at breakfast and then drink 2 glasses of water. It's great for providing fibre.

+ Magnesium.

+ Vitamin D to help prevent osteoporosis, colon and breast cancer.

If you've tried all the advice for a month and your condition still hasn't improved then see your doctor first. You may also want to subsequently consult a nutritionist.

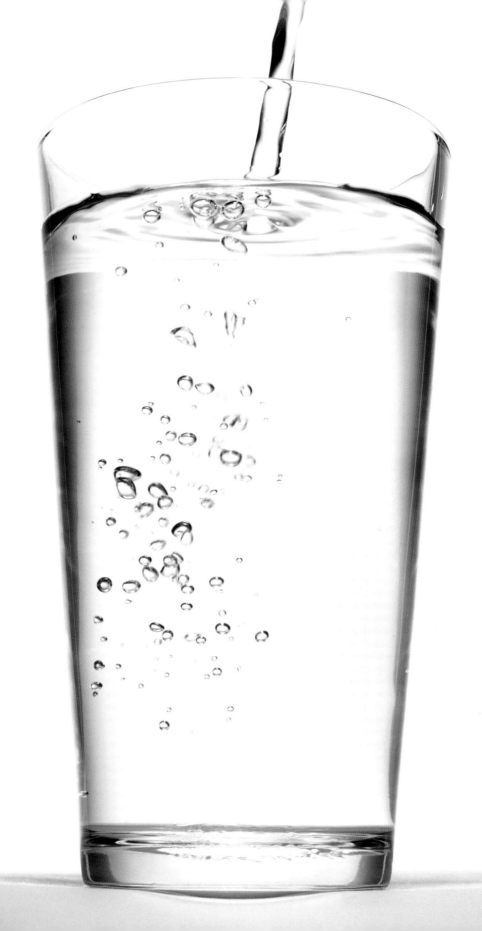

Diverticulosis

As 80 per cent of people with diverticulosis have no symptoms at all, most people discover that they have it when they have an acute attack of pain the stomach or when they go for a test on their colon for other reasons. This is despite the fact that it is a common condition over the age of 50, caused for the most part by constipation and a low fibre diet, and aggravated by obesity, stress and smoking. Straining to pass hard stools causes increased pressure on the colon's walls, which then develop weak areas or blow outs that produce tiny sacs or diverticuli. Once they develop they don't go away.

Symptoms may include cramping and gas, and pain on the left side of the stomach that is relieved by passing a bowel movement. Occasionally the diverticuli bleed, causing bright red blood on the stool, or block sometimes causing pain and fever. In all of these situations you should consult with your doctor but you may also be helped by the action plan below.

Diverticulosis action plan

During an acute attack of diverticulosis, when the bowel is inflamed:

+ Make some cabbage soup. Cabbage is rich in glutamine, a fantastic help in healing the gut lining and providing fuel to the intestinal cells.

+ Add ginger when cooking or drink ginger tea as it soothes and heals the gut.

+ Use lots of garlic when cooking as this is a wonderful natural antibiotic.

+ Reduce your intake of high-fibre grains, particularly the wheat bran in cereals, as these can be abrasive to the gut wall. Gradually eat more of them as you recover.

+ Cook vegetables in soup and don't eat salad, which is hard to digest and has too much fibre. As you improve, move on to lightly steamed vegetables.

+ Don't eat fresh fruit but opt for apple sauce or lightly stewed pears or apricots.

+ If you are on antibiotics then avoid yeast and sugar for 2 weeks as these will promote the overgrowth of yeast in the gut. Take live plain natural yoghurt and acidophilus capsules for a month to provide good bowel bacteria.

+ Aloe vera juice is wonderfully healing, as is slippery elm. Drink for 2 weeks.

+ Try to stop smoking and reduce your stress levels.

+ Avoid food that can get lodged in the sacs such as grape seeds, sweetcorn and nuts. Also reduce red meat as this has a low transit time.

Prevention is better than the cure so follow the Constipation action plan on page 71 to avoid diverticulosis.

Food intolerance

It's a cruel fact that many people are intolerant to the very food they crave. And sometimes it's not just junk food that's bad for you – ironically, the good fresh stuff you're eating might also be making you feel unwell. A food intolerance is caused by your immune system reacting against a particular food – a reaction sparked off by something in your genes, your diet or early environment. Wheat and dairy are the most common food intolerances, but almost any food or foods may affect an individual. The problem is that intolerances produce a range of symptoms that could easily be attributed to other causes: digestive upsets, weight problems, recurrent respiratory infections, fluid retention, excess mucus in the nose, throat and sinuses, frequent urination, mouth ulcers, depression, fatigue, muscle pains, palpitations – a host of usually low-level, everyday ailments.

If you identify a number of recurring symptoms like these, say five, and the suggestions in this book don't improve them, it's worth testing yourself for food intolerances.

Food intolerances change and so just because you have tested positive for one food now does not mean to say that you are going to be sensitive to it for the rest of your life, particularly if it is a mild intolerance. With mild intolerances it is always worth reintroducing the food every fourth day after a few months and seeing how the body copes with it. Only reintroduce one new food at a time.

The focus here is on food intolerances, not the classic allergies that are much rarer and cause severe symptoms like constricted airways and grossly swollen eyes – think of peanuts and anaphylactic shock. Such cases need professional assessment and specific advice.

✚ Food intolerance test

This is a simple test that you can do on your own, but you have to buy a special kit to do so. All you have to do is to collect some blood from a pin prick and draw it up into a tiny tube, which you post with a form to the lab. Within two weeks you'll be sent a report telling you which foods you are mildly, moderately and very sensitive to.

For further details on where to buy this kit, see page 218.

Irritable bowel syndrome

Irritable bowel syndrome (IBS) is a persistent disorder associated with gas, bloating, abdominal pain and diarrhoea alternating with constipation, for which, historically no cause has been found. It's thought to be due to a nervous disorder and was in the past called spastic colon. However, the symptoms may well have other causes, such as:

+ Poor diet.

+ Food intolerances.

+ Too much caffeine and alcohol.

+ Lack of digestive enzymes.

+ An undiagnosed parasite infection.

+ Overgrowth of yeast following the use of antibiotics or the contraceptive pill.

+ Too little good bowel bacteria and too many unhealthy bacteria. (A study done at the Gastrointestinal motility program at Cedars-Sinai Medical Centre in Beverly Hills, California in 2000 found that 78% of people with IBS had bacterial overgrowth in the small intestine.)

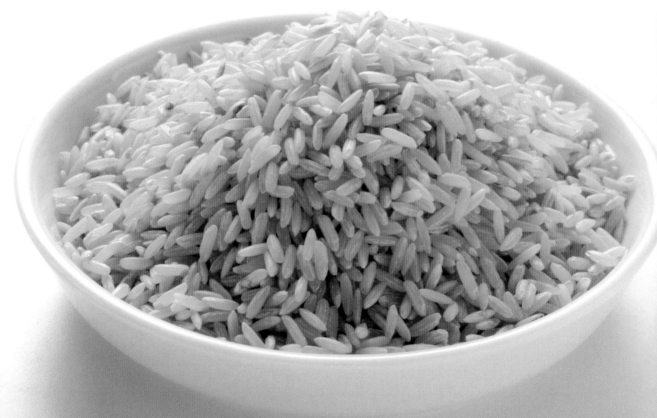

IBS action plan

Dr Wendy says: 'In my experience, relatively few people have the true irritable bowel syndrome. As many as 60 per cent of my patients with comparable gut symptoms (where other diagnoses have been ruled out) have benefited from the following recommendations:

- Eat a high-fibre diet including 6 to 8 helpings of fresh fruit and vegetables per day, and whole grains, particularly brown rice.

- Take adequate protein in the form of fish, organic chicken and tofu.

- Avoid spicy food, coffee and smoking, all of which irritate the gut.

- Chew your food well.

- Take natural yogurt without sugar (not a yogurt drink) to increase bowel flora. Along with this you may want to take a good acidophilus supplement daily.

- Reduce sugar to the occasional piece of chocolate.

- Drink 6 to 8 glasses of water per day, but not more than one glass at meal times.

- Reduce alcohol, particularly wine, beer and champagne which irritate the lining of the colon and may promote a yeast imbalance.

- Stop drinking all carbonated drinks.

'Try these steps with the supplements for a month. If you still have symptoms, then see a nutritionist or a doctor who specialises in nutritional medicine. If you're not improving after two months on this regime, then consult your GP.'

Supplements for IBS

- Aloe vera juice is great for healing the lining of the gut, but do not drink it if your stools are loose because it is a natural laxative.

- Psyllium or linseeds are a great source of fibre so take if constipated.

- To relieve bloating you may want to take peppermint capsules or tea after meals.

- Glutamine powder helps to heal the lining of the gut.

- A good multivitamin and mineral will supply those nutrients lost or not absorbed.

- Magnesium taken in the evening, particularly if you are more prone to stress. Take aspartate or malate if you have a loose stool.

- The other thing worth having handy is Buscopan, an anti-spasmodic that can relieve gut-wrenching cramps. It is a prescription drug so you must get it from your doctor.

digestion

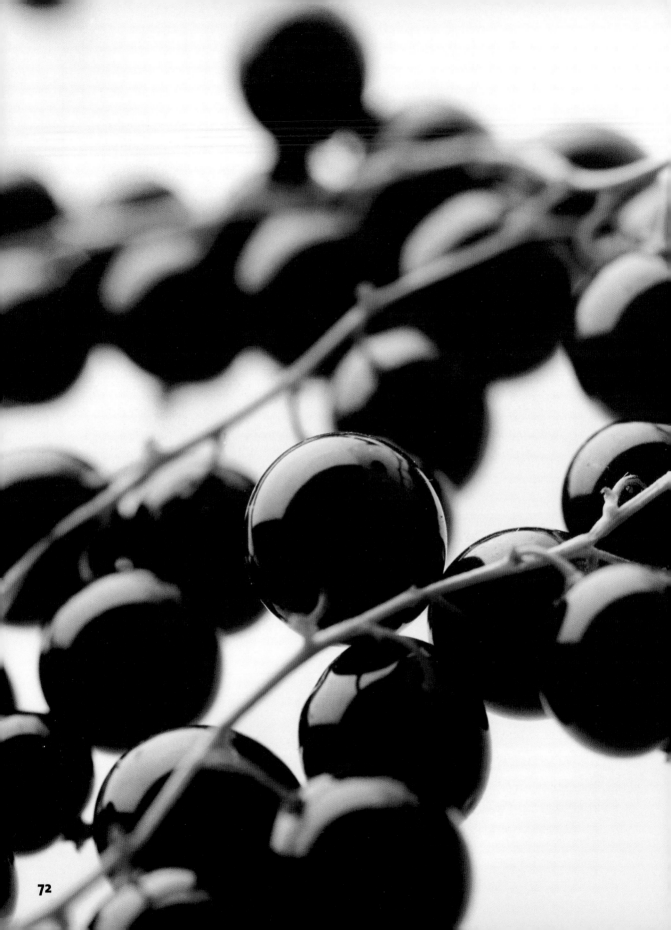

Haemorrhoids/piles

Piles are formed when the veins just inside the anus become enlarged – they're like varicose veins, only in the canal of the anus, not the legs. The commonest cause is straining with bowel movements, but they also occur frequently in pregnancy, in obese people and those who don't exercise. The symptoms tend to depend on where the piles are, but may include bright red blood when wiping after a stool, itching, burning, or a swelling outside the anus. Internal piles, inside the anal canal, tend to give bright red bleeding but no pain. External piles, which are just at the opening of the anal canal, can also bleed but more often cause itching and burning and form a lump.

 ## Haemorrhoids action plan

Prevention is definitely better than cure with piles. The best way to do this is to avoid constipation and straining to pass your stools (see the action plan on page 66 – you'll also benefit from eating foods rich in bioflavonoids, like berries, cherries and citrus fruit). Don't forget that sometimes it may be the medication you're taking that is making you constipated, such as iron tablets, antacids and antidepressants.

✛ Once your piles have cleared up, you can help prevent them recurring by washing with cold water after each bowel movement, and taking psyllium to soften your stool.

✛ Although the commonest cause of fresh red bleeding from the bowel is piles, it's always advisable to visit the doctor to rule out any serious condition.

 ## Supplements for piles

For the acute phase:

✛ Bromelain is a natural anti-inflammatory.

✛ Vitamin C and bioflavonoid to help heal and strengthen tissue.

✛ Horse-chestnut capsules to help strengthen capillaries.

✛ Calendula or vitamin E cream applied topically will reduce soreness, as will aloe vera gel.

For the chronic phase, see supplements for constipation on page 66.

Gallbladder and gallstones

Have you ever had an acute attack of pain in the right upper part of the abdomen after eating a very fatty meal? If so, you may well be suffering with gallstones and have just had a gallbladder attack.

The gallbladder is a small pear-shaped organ situated underneath the liver. It stores bile, which has been produced by the liver and released to digest fat in the duodenum. If the gallbladder isn't working properly, then you can have a problem with digesting fats. This can lead to gallstones, which are very common and increase with age and obesity. They form when the bile is either too thick or not flowing freely. The commonest cause is when the liver produces bile that has too much cholesterol in it, which is generally due to:

+ A high-cholesterol diet
+ Obesity
+ Excessive intake of refined carbohydrates
+ High oestrogen levels
+ Cholesterol-lowering drugs

As a result of the association with high oestrogen levels, women are twice as likely as men to have gallstones, particularly if they are obese, have had multiple pregnancies or are on the contraceptive pill. In fact, gallstones were traditionally linked to being 'fair, fat, female and forty'. This is no longer true – gallstones are being diagnosed in younger people, partly because of the widespread use of the contraceptive pill and partly because of diets commonly high in fat and refined carbohydrate.

If gallstones get stuck on their way to the duodenum and prevent bile being released, the pressure will build up and an infection may be caused. That's when things get serious – you'll need prompt hospital treatment that may even lead to removing the gallbladder. It's much better to prevent gallstones forming in the first place – or, if you've had them, prevent them recurring, with a healthier diet and lifestyle that is the basis for good health generally.

80% of gallstones are made of solid cholesterol. They can be any size from a pea to a golf ball

Gallstones action plan

+ Exercise regularly.

+ Increase dietary fibre by eating more vegetables, fruit and wholegrains.

+ Eat a diet low in saturated fats.

+ Lose weight.

Supplements for gallstones

+ Vitamin C

+ Omega-3 and 6 essential fatty acids, found in hempseed oil

+ Lecithin capsule or granules, which help to emulsify cholesterol

+ Digestive enzymes containing lipase with each meal

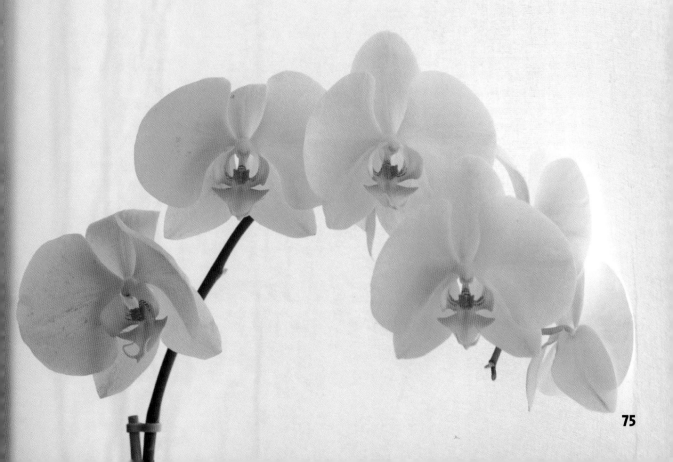

Heartburn

Heartburn is a burning sensation in the stomach and/or chest. For some people the pain is so severe it can feel like a heart attack. It is caused by the sphincter muscle between the stomach and the oesophagus not closing properly, allowing food and acid to travel back from the stomach into the oesophagus. This oesophageal tissue was not designed for acid and the pain you feel is literally the burning pain of acid on sensitive tissue.

As heartburn is more likely to be related to the mechanics of the oesophagus, stomach and gastro-oesophegal sphincter muscle rather than to stomach acid levels alone, people with both high and low stomach acid levels can be affected by heartburn. People who have low stomach acid do not empty their stomachs as quickly so there is more food in the upper part of the stomach which then puts pressure on the sphincter to open, leading to acid reflux. Overweight people can also suffer from the condition as excess stomach fat can affect the workings of the sphincter, as does eating too much or too quickly. A recent study showed that reflux occurred more often when a standard meal is eaten fast in five minutes compared with the same meal eaten slowly over 30 minutes.

So before you reach for your favourite antacid look at the Heartburn action plan and see what you can change.

 ## Heartburn action plan

+ Stop smoking.

+ Reduce your alcohol intake.

+ Chew your food slowly and well.

+ Eat small, regular meals.

+ Reduce your weight so that your BMI (see page 14) is 25 or less.

+ Avoid eating late so that your stomach is not full when you go to bed.

+ Avoid bending after meals.

+ Sleep in a slightly raised position to prevent stomach contents coming back into the oesophagus.

+ Eat more zinc-rich food – eggs, pumpkin seeds, almonds, oysters and turkey – to help repair the tissues.

+ Follow the stomach acid action plan on page 66.

   QUICK TIP: At the first sign of heartburn, drink one or two large glasses of water. This may relieve the heartburn by washing the acid out of the oesophagus.

Another condition commonly associated with heartburn is hiatus hernia. Normally the whole of the stomach lies in the abdominal cavity below the diaphragm, but when you have a hiatus hernia then a small part of the stomach pushes up in the oesophageal opening and ends up in the chest. This alteration in pressure means that the sphincter may not always be able to close efficiently and so acid reflux may follow. Drinking alcohol and smoking also cause the sphincter to relax and so are more likely to cause heartburn.

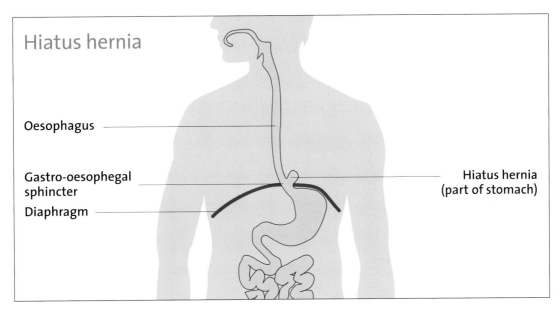

However just because you have a hiatus hernia does not mean that you will have reflux. The people who are the most troubled are those with the large hernias. For the others, up to 50 per cent of people will have a hernia but only a few will have persistent symptoms.

Supplements for heartburn

+ **Aloe vera taken daily will heal the lining of the gut**
+ **Slippery elm also helps the gut lining**
+ **Zinc picolinate**

Reflux occurs more often when a meal is eaten fast. Eat slowly for thirty minutes, not quickly for five

The liver

The miracle organ! Most of us know that our liver is important but haven't a clue what it does, apart from breaking down alcohol.

In fact the liver is one of the most important organs in the body. It's the largest solid organ, weighing over 2 kilos (5 pounds) and using no less than 12 per cent of your total energy supply. The body can function without the stomach or colon but not without the liver.

In traditional Chinese medicine, the health of the liver is considered representative of the whole body; if your liver is healthy then you are healthy. Conditions such as depression, anxiety, hormone balances, poor digestion and headaches, to name a few, are treated by improving liver health.

One of the unique features of the liver is its dual blood supply. The portal vein carries blood and all its nutrients from the intestine, the stomach and spleen. Alongside this, the hepatic artery enters the liver bringing blood from the rest of the body – as much as a pint of blood can be held in the liver at any one time. Within the liver these two blood vessels divide into tree-like structures, getting progressively smaller and smaller. The tiniest branches end in the liver lobules or cells, which are where the two different bloods mix and all the many biochemical processes go on.

What overworks the liver:

+ Alcohol

+ Prescription drugs

+ Recreational drugs

+ Exposure to toxic chemicals (e.g. pesticides, herbicides, paints)

+ Improper digestion

+ Toxic bowel

+ Hypothyroid

+ Repressed emotion

+ Smoking (tobacco and marijuana)

And specifically where diet is concerned:

+ Overeating

+ Excess refined carbohydrates, especially sugar

+ Excess processed fats, especially fried food

+ Fast food or junk food

+ Low fibre intake

+ Not enough fruit and vegetables

+ Eating when stressed or rushed

What the liver does

The liver is extraordinarily complex – it has over 500 known functions, which are divided into four main areas:

1 Detoxification

The liver neutralises toxins that come to it from the lungs, the bowel and the skin, such as drugs, hormones, alcohol, toxic chemicals, bacteria and viruses and allergens.

It's a two-step process. The first step can actually make the toxin more poisonous before it's broken down in the second phase. If the liver is overloaded, some of the toxic substance will not make it to the second stage immediately and may accumulate – which is why you want to avoid overloading your liver with, for example, excessive amounts of alcohol. If it is overburdened, then hormones such as oestrogen may accumulate, causing higher circulating levels of hormones. This is why high alcohol consumption may be associated with breast cancer.

Food for thought, though, is that one of the most challenging burdens for the liver is breaking down the large number of chemicals produced by stress!

2 Production

Every day the liver makes many of the clotting factors in the blood, as well as a number of substances that are vital for the proper functioning of the body: bile, cholesterol, albumin, lymph and gamma globulins.

3 Conversion

The liver provides a critical function in processing most of our food. It converts glycogen, a highly concentrated storage form of carbohydrate, to glucose and vice versa. By doing this, the liver plays a very important role in blood sugar control, releasing sugar when necessary and storing it again when it is not required.

The liver also converts fat into forms that the body can use, and produces 60 per cent of the usable energy made from fat in the diet. Protein is built up into the complex proteins required by the blood and immune system – albumin and globulin. It can also be converted into glucose for the body.

4 Storage

The liver stores blood, vitamins A, D, E, K, B12, iron and glycogen. Stored vitamin D can last four months, and vitamin B12 can last up to two years.

The liver has to break down the large number of chemicals produced by stress

A sluggish liver

When the liver is overburdened, it can't properly filter poisons out of the blood. One of the first places that this shows up is the skin – which is also important in eliminating waste – causing acne and rashes. And as the liver is vital for the immune system, you will be more prone to coughs, colds and other infections, as well as allergies.

Signs of a sluggish liver

+ Fatigue
+ Nausea
+ Mood swings and Irritability
+ Bloating

+ Raised cholesterol
+ Skin rashes or acne
+ Coated or puffy sides of tongue
+ Dark circles under the eyes

+ Intolerance to fatty foods
+ Menstrual irregularities
+ Difficulty losing weight
+ Obesity/overweight

Furthermore, the whole metabolism will become sluggish, making it very difficult to lose weight in this state. So, to improve your health and to actually lose weight, it's vital to improve the liver so that it can do its job of detoxification and improve the body's metabolic functioning.

What happens to drugs

As the blood and all its constituents are first processed through the liver before reaching the rest of the body, drugs or hormones taken orally may be broken down by 90 per cent before they even have a chance to work in the body as a whole. For this reason, hormones or drugs are sometimes given under the tongue, on the skin, or vaginally or rectally, so that they can enter the body and be immediately effective. A lower dose can then be used and the liver may be spared a lot of extra work.

It also means that the amount of drug that actually reaches the body depends on how well the liver is working. For instance, if you're on the contraceptive pill and you drink a lot of alcohol one night, then your body will process the pill quite differently from the way it would if you had just gone on a liver cleanse.

Non-alcoholic fatty liver disease

Alcohol probably gets the most blame for liver disease since most people know it kills liver cells. Too much of it – a steady intake of four or more drinks a day for men and three or more drinks a day for women – can cause what is called fatty liver disease. But there's another condition that is not induced by alcohol, called, unsurprisingly, non-alcoholic fatty liver disease.

This is rapidly becoming the most common chronic liver condition in the western world. Although it is found in all age groups it is most often diagnosed in middle-aged women who are overweight or obese, and who have metabolic syndrome. This is closely associated with resistance to insulin (the hormone that regulates blood sugar) in which fat gets abnormally laid down in the liver cells due to the body's inability to cope with glucose and fat (see page 99).

The true incidence of non-alcoholic fatty liver disease is as yet unknown because it is a relatively new diagnosis, but some people believe that it affects at least a third of American adults.

Most cases of the disease will remain stable for many years causing little serious harm, albeit contributing to a sluggish liver and overall lack of optimum health. Ten per cent of people will go on to develop serious disease such as cirrhosis, caused by a second hit to the liver such as a viral infection or moderate alcohol consumption.

The lack of early-warning symptoms means that the disease is usually found when you go to the doctor to have liver tests, which are then found to be abnormal. If there are any symptoms, they tend to be non-specific, including fatigue, malaise, or a dull ache in the upper right of the abdomen.

As the liver is so vital for the immune system a sluggish liver will contribute to coughs, colds, infections and allergies

digestion

Liver action plan

+ Diet and exercise

The most effective diet is one rich in fibre and low in saturated fats, with 6 to 8 servings of fruit and vegetables a day, and reduced intake of animal fats and dairy foods. Eat foods high in vitamin E (such as seeds, peas and sardines) and vitamin C (such as green leafy vegetables and tomatoes). Eat oily fish such as salmon, herrings and sardines, which are good sources of omega-3 fatty acids. Stop taking sugar or sugar substitutes of any sort because fluctuations in blood sugar can, even if you're not diabetic, lead to you converting sugar into fat, which is then deposited in the liver. Accordingly, you should also take no alcohol or caffeine.

To complement this essential diet regime, you should have a good aerobic exercise session for half an hour four times per week.

+ Diabetes control

If you're diabetic, the condition needs to be managed strictly with diet, medications or insulin to keep blood sugar levels stable. This will also help to prevent further liver damage and reduce the amount of accumulated fat in the liver.

+ Cholesterol control

If you have raised levels of cholesterol and triglycerides, these need to be brought back into the normal range. This is best done by diet and exercise initially. If this isn't enough then consider medication or supplements to lower your cholesterol.

+ Avoidance of toxic substances

As well as alcohol, you need to avoid any medications that can damage the liver. You may wish to talk to your doctor to see if your medication should be changed. And don't forget the danger of exposure to synthetic chemicals such as those in household cleaning products, pesticide residues in food, and junk food – the liver must process many new chemicals, and too little is known about their combined effect.

If you have a sluggish liver, consultation with a good nutritionist can be extremely beneficial.

Supplements for the liver

+ Milk thistle

+ Omega-3 fatty acids or flaxseed oil – take fat to lose fat!

+ A good multivitamin and mineral

+ Coenzyme Q10

the diet doctors inside and out

The pancreas

Most people have heard about the pancreas in relation to diabetes – which is what you'll get if the pancreas packs up. In fact the pancreatic cells have two functions: 99 per cent of them produce the daily 1,500ml of pancreatic juice that is poured into the small intestine to neutralise stomach acid and to help digestion. The remaining 1 per cent produce insulin, glucagon and other hormones that help balance your blood sugar. It is when these cells can no longer produce enough insulin to keep pace with the body's demands that diabetes develops.

Like the liver, the pancreas itself can be badly affected by obesity, excessive alcohol, and a poor diet high in sugars and fats. It's yet another case of prevention being infinitely better than cure.

In traditional Chinese medicine, the health of the liver is considered representative of the whole body; if your liver is healthy then you are healthy

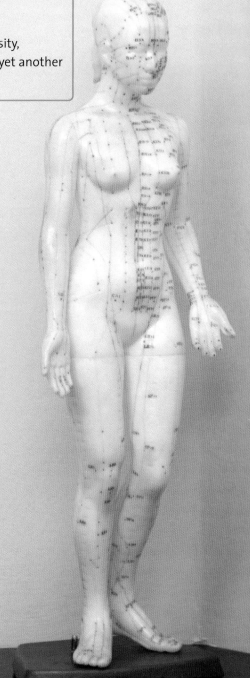

Hormones and metabolism
The balancing act

Hormones are the body's chemical messengers circulating in the bloodstream. They ebb and flow with the body's changing needs and have a profound effect on our emotional and physical wellbeing. In a delicate balancing act, hormones work on many different parts of the body at the same time. Their effects last for hours, days, months, even years. That balance has to be maintained for good all-round health, while for effective weight loss you need to know the role of the major hormones involved.

Know your glands

Hormones are secreted by the endocrine glands, which are found in various parts of the body. These are controlled by the main gland, the pituitary, in the base of the brain. In turn, the pituitary is controlled by chemical and electrical messages from a part of the brain called the hypothalamus.

The glands of major relevance here are: the ovaries and testes which, naturally, produce sex hormones; the thyroid, whose hormones control metabolism; the adrenal glands which produce hormones that regulate stress, water and mineral balance and some sex hormones; and the pancreas whose hormones regulate blood sugar levels.

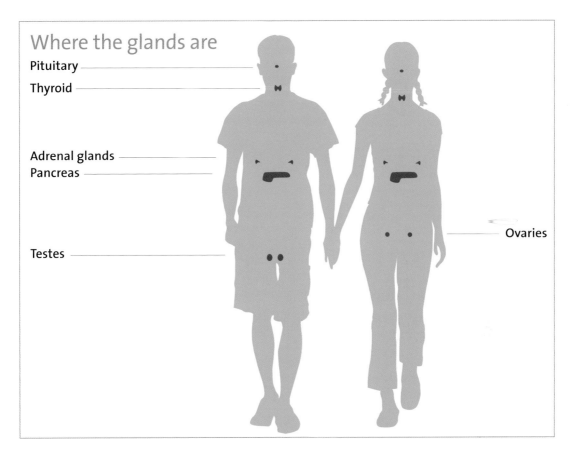

Where the glands are

Pituitary
Thyroid
Adrenal glands
Pancreas
Testes
Ovaries

Balancing female hormones

The ovary, which produces oestrogen, progesterone and testosterone, is so called for its essential function of producing ova (eggs). Oestrogen stimulates egg production, and prepares the lining of the uterus for pregnancy. In the middle of the menstrual cycle, the egg is released and then either fertilised by sperm or not. If it isn't fertilised, then it becomes what is called the corpus luteum, which secretes the other main female hormone, progesterone, for the next 14 days until it dies. As it dies, levels of oestrogen and progesterone fall, and the uterus lining is shed, producing the next period. And so the cycle continues.

For a woman to have good hormonal health, her oestrogen and progesterone need to be in dynamic balance; so, whether she is planning to become pregnant or not, ovulation is important. The balance may be disturbed from time to time, for a variety of reasons, but most commonly through stress. The system can cope with some disruption but, if it happens repeatedly, it may set up irregular and/or heavy bleeding cycles due to a pattern called oestrogen dominance (see overleaf). Furthermore, an overweight or obese woman is less likely to ovulate and more likely to have higher circulating levels of oestrogen because of a sluggish liver not breaking down the hormones quickly (see page 80), creating even more likelihood of oestrogen dominance, contributing to uterine fibroids, endometriosis and PMS.

Features of oestrogen dominance

+ Weight gain, with fat deposited especially at hips and thighs

+ Water retention

+ Breast swelling

+ Premenstrual syndrome

+ Depression and/or mood swings

+ Loss of libido

+ Heavy or irregular bleeding

+ Craving for sweets

 ## Oestrogen dominance action plan

+ Reduce exposure to xeno-oestrogens (i.e. hormones found in the environment – as in pesticides, plastics and household chemicals).

+ Eat phyto-oestrogens, found in soyabeans, tofu, miso, beansprouts, sunflower seeds, chickpeas, lentils and many fruits and vegetables.

+ Increase fibre intake through fruits, vegetables and whole grains, especially oats. Oestrogen, once it has been used by the cells, is processed by the liver and binds to fibre in the intestines for excretion. If there is no fibre, it is recirculated in the body.

+ Eat organic produce whenever possible, particularly red meat, dairy and chicken, all of which have been shown to contain hormones if non-organic.

+ Reduce alcohol intake, which the liver breaks down before oestrogen – leading to recycling of the hormone.

+ Keep bowel flora healthy. Unhealthy bacteria in the gut will 'unhook' oestrogen from fibre so it is not excreted.

+ Avoid constipation – women with smaller stools have been shown to have increased levels of oestrogen. Constipated women are also more likely to have pre-cancerous cells in their breasts. Vegetarian women with a high fibre, low-animal fat diet have a lower incidence of breast cancer than meat eaters.

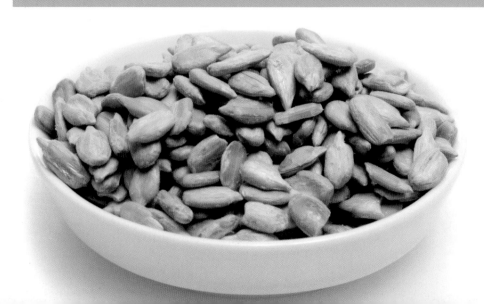

Polycystic Ovary Syndrome

Are you having difficulty losing weight? Do you suffer with acne and have irregular periods? If so, then you may be suffering from polycystic ovary syndrome (PCOS). This is a condition in which cysts develop on your ovaries. It is increasingly common, perhaps because of its strong association with excess body fat, and it's now being diagnosed in 5–10 per cent of women of childbearing age.

The major problems with polycystic ovaries are that a woman's eggs do not develop properly and her body produces too many hormones known as androgens. Androgens, like testosterone, are produced by the ovaries and the adrenal glands, but in women with PCOS they are present in much higher levels than normal, often because of high levels of circulating insulin.

Why this is the case is not clear, but it is known that PCOS is strongly associated with excess body fat (50 per cent of women with the condition are overweight), which in turn is associated with higher levels of circulating insulin. This is particularly so if you have a high waist-to-hip ratio (the so-called apple shape, see page 165).

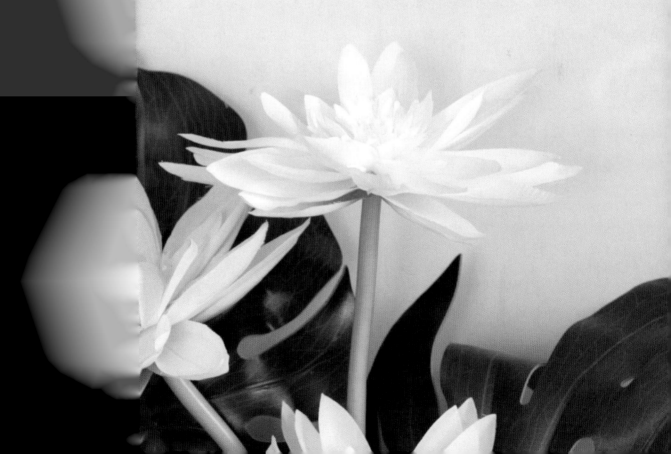

Polycystic ovaries now affect 1 in 10 women

Chronic high levels of androgens upset a woman's normal hormonal cycle, which in turn blocks the growth and development of eggs. As a result her ovaries may contain many small cysts from underdeveloped eggs. She frequently will not ovulate and so progesterone levels are low. High testosterone levels also lead to acne and excess body hair. Features of PCOS include:

+ Being overweight or finding it difficult to lose weight
+ Acne
+ Excess body hair
+ Irregular periods with longer cycle length
+ Infertility

High circulating levels of insulin and androgens lead to an increased risk for obesity, diabetes, heart disease and hypertension. To test for PCOS visit your doctor who will probably want to order blood tests to check your hormone, sugar and cholesterol levels. The diagnostic test is an ultrasound of the pelvis, which will show the multiple cysts on the surface of the ovary.

PCOS action plan

+ The main thing to appreciate is that it can be difficult to lose weight, but doing so is critical to treating this condition and preventing the long-term consequences. If you are one of the lucky ones with a normal weight, you may be at higher risk of getting hypoglycaemia because of the increased circulating levels of insulin.

+ The key to weight loss is balancing your blood sugar levels to lower insulin levels and exercising to increase insulin sensitivity. For more information on this see the exercise section on page 188.

Supplements for PCOS

+ Chromium to help balance blood sugar
+ Zinc for making insulin
+ Saw palmetto may be helpful for reducing body hair
+ Good multivitamin and mineral supplements for general well-being

Balancing male hormones

The balance of hormones is equally important to men. Just as women have some testosterone in their system, so men have some oestrogen. Again, when the balance is disturbed, as particularly in the case of obese men, the effect can be far-reaching.

Obese men with pot bellies are likely to develop breast tissue. This is because fat is actually a hormonal gland and fat tissues in the abdomen convert testosterone into oestrogens. At the same time as obese men are getting raised levels of oestrogen, they're not making as much testosterone because of the foods they eat – a study has shown that eating a meal high in saturated fat reduced testosterone levels for up to four hours. On the other hand, protein and high-carbohydrate meals had no such effect.

So it appears that obese men can get testosterone deficiency as a result of the abdominal fat cells, and also from the fat they eat. The resulting hormone imbalance of too much oestrogen and not enough free testosterone partially explains why so many men in this condition are impotent and experience a wide range of premature degenerative diseases, as well as the threat of cardiovascular disease (see page 44) and type-2 diabetes (see page 99).

 ## Male hormone action plan

+ Lose weight as a priority.

+ Reduce all saturated fat in the diet.

+ Eat high-protein food – organic chicken, eggs, fish, tofu, beans and lentils – at least twice a day.

+ Eat plenty of fruit and vegetables to provide antioxidants to support the body as fat is broken down. Fat contains many toxic chemicals which, when released, can produce free radicals (thought to be responsible for a lot of degenerative conditions in the body) which must be minimised by high antioxidant intake.

+ Avoid alcohol as it acts like the fat cells to increase oestrogen and lower testosterone.

+ Increase your exercise pattern gradually until you are doing at least four sessions a week for 30 minutes.

Eating the wrong fats lowers your testosterone levels – and sex drive

The thyroid

If you're feeling tired, tend to feel the cold and are having a lot of difficulty losing weight, then you may have a sluggish thyroid. The thyroid is a small butterfly-shaped gland, sitting just below your voice box. Regulating the body's metabolism, it determines the temperature of the body and the speed at which it burns calories or fuel. So the thyroid is essentially your fat-burning gland.

The thyroid makes two main hormones, known in their short form as T4 and T3. These need iodine, zinc and selenium to function, so it's important to make sure you have enough of these minerals. As the thyroid has an impact on every cell in the body, if it is underactive then you will have a variety of symptoms, including:

+ Cold hands and feet
+ Tendency to feel the cold
+ Fatigue, particularly in the mornings
+ Depression
+ Dry skin

+ Headaches
+ Constipation
+ Diffuse loss of hair
+ Aching in the joints
+ Muscle cramps in the feet at night

+ Swollen eyelids (especially in the morning)
+ Swelling in hands and feet
+ Heavy or irregular periods
+ Infertility
+ Loss of libido, or impotence

In general terms, low levels of thyroid hormone lead to retention of water, salt and protein in the body. Nails, skin and hair will grow slowly. Cholesterol levels in the blood will go up. The thyroid is intimately connected with other hormones, which may, therefore, also be affected.

If you suffer with three or more of the symptoms in the above list, including, most importantly, feeling the cold all the time, it would be a good idea to test yourself at home (see box opposite). Diagnosis is confirmed by blood tests (which should include cholesterol) taken by your doctor.

A small percentage of patients who have an underactive thyroid have been found to have an intolerance to wheat and have improved when that has been removed from their diets. If your blood tests do not confirm a thyroid problem but you have three or more of the symptoms, then correct any mineral deficiency and follow the action plan opposite.

Exercising regularly will help your thyroid work more effectively

✚ Tests for underactive thyroid

Generally speaking, a low body temperature reflects an under-functioning thyroid. Use a mercury thermometer, and prepare it the night before by shaking it down and keeping it by your bed. When you wake in the morning, put the thermometer under your arm and stay lying down for 10 minutes (don't get out of bed until the 10 minutes are up). Remove the thermometer and read it immediately. Repeat the test on five consecutive mornings.

Pre-menopausal women need to do this test in the first 5–7 days of the cycle (before the temperature rises with the cycle). Post-menopausal women and men can take their temperature any day.

The normal body temperature in the morning is 36.6–36.8°C. A temperature of 36.4°C or lower suggests a sluggish thyroid.

In addition, as iodine, zinc and selenium aid the function of the thyroid, test to make sure you are not deficient in these minerals (see page 39).

Thyroid action plan

- ✚ Make sure you are getting enough iodine in your diet by eating seaweed (including kelp), seafood and garlic.

- ✚ Keep your selenium levels up by eating lots of hummus, brown and green lentils, mushrooms, sunflower and sesame seeds, cashew and brazil nuts.

- ✚ Eat zinc-rich foods such as almonds, quorn, tofu, oysters, crab, chicken, turkey and pumpkin seeds.

- ✚ Take wheat out of your diet for a month and see if you have better energy levels.

- ✚ Exercise can help the thyroid to work more effectively.

Supplements for underactive thyroid

- ✚ Kelp
- ✚ Selenium
- ✚ Zinc
- ✚ A multivitamin and mineral, geared to the thyroid
- ✚ Flaxseed oil

Hormones and stress

'Stress' seems to be a catch-all term for almost anything that makes us feel enough pressure to be anxious, from the truly serious to the seemingly trivial. Strictly speaking, stress is defined as a reaction to a physical, mental or emotional stimulus that upsets the body's natural balance. This could apply to most of us some of the time, or even all of the time.

Our bodies must have evolved to cope with stress, but the peculiar, possibly unprecedented, kinds of stress that modern life inflicts on us do seem to have adverse consequences on the body, in both the short term and the long term. Most people recognise some things that cause stress in their lives, such as a busy work load, overdue bills, traffic, traffic wardens etc. But some of the things people don't recognise as stress inducers are:

+ Lack of sleep

+ Excessive alcohol consumption

+ Smoking

+ Blood sugar imbalances

+ Nutrient deficiencies

+ Food allergies and intolerances

+ Medicines and hormone imbalances

+ A poorly functioning bowel leading to toxic waste build-up

The adrenal glands are primarily responsible for producing the hormones caused by stress. Sitting on top of the kidneys, they have two distinct parts, the adrenal cortex which makes up 85 per cent of the gland, and the adrenal medulla. The adrenal cortex produces: cortisol, which regulates metabolism and resistance to stress; aldosterone which helps regulate salt and water balance; and androgens, the most important of which is DHEA (Dehydroepiandrosterone) which can be metabolised in the body to testosterone, oestrogen and other androgens. The adrenal medulla produces adrenalin and noradrenalin which are released in times of stress.

In the acute phase, the familiar 'fight or flight' response causes adrenalin and noradrenalin to be released, putting the body into a heightened state of awareness. Longer term stress, on the other hand, is predominantly mediated by the hormone cortisol and it is the persistently elevated levels of cortisol that takes the toll on the body, causing:

+ Raised cholesterol levels

+ Hypoglycaemia (low blood sugar levels, see page 96)

+ Insulin resistance

+ Weight gain

+ Lowered immunity leading to more frequent colds and infections

+ Increased risk of osteoporosis as cortisol stimulates the cells that break down bone

+ Weakness and pain, caused by the muscles losing their ability to take up glucose efficiently

Stress responses

This table shows how our bodies react to stress and the symptoms these reactions create in us, both in the short and the long term.

Stress response	Associated symptoms
The heart rate increases to pump extra blood around the body to get oxygen and vital nutrients to the cells.	Rapid or irregular heartbeats.
Breathing becomes more rapid to allow more oxygen into the body.	Rapid ventilation rate and asthma.
Blood pressure goes up, triggered by stress hormones.	High blood pressure.
Stress hormones are released, usually adrenalin and noradrenalin from the adrenal glands.	High blood pressure, panic, anxiety and anger.
The liver releases stored glucose into the blood to provide more energy.	Panic and anxiety.
Blood is directed towards the brain and muscles carrying increased quantities of oxygen, glucose and nutrients.	High blood pressure, migraine and headaches.
Blood is directed away from the surface of skin in hands and feet.	Cold hands and feet and sexual dysfunction.
Blood is directed away from the digestive and reproductive organs because, for immediate survival, digesting food and sex are a low priority.	Upset stomach, increased colitis, constipation, poor digestion of foods, infertility.
Perspiration. The body perspires to cool the body's increased metabolism.	Excess sweating and dehydration.
Heightened senses for survival vigilance. We become more sensitive to noise, light, smell and touch. The thinking part of the brain partially shuts down and the survival mechanisms in the middle and lower, more primitive, parts of the brain take over so we react to things rather than thinking them through. Basic emotions such as fear, anger, sadness, joy and depression take over.	Dilated pupils, irritability, anxiety, depression, poor impulse control, poor problem solving, reduced communication abilities and increased substance abuse.

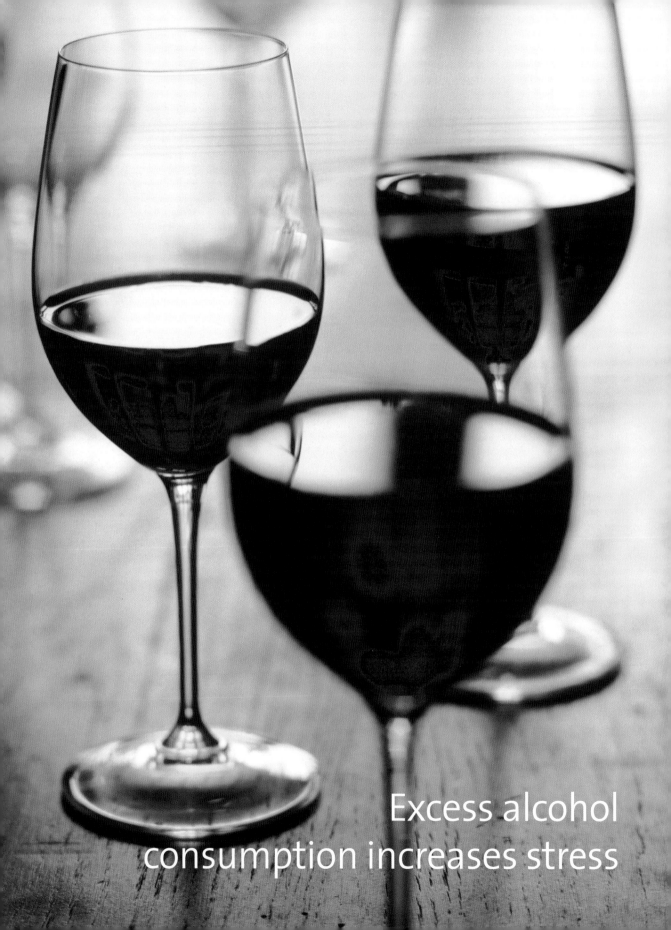

Excess alcohol
consumption increases stress

Stress reduction action plan

Stress is an external and an internal experience. You can reduce your external stimuli by changing certain elements in your lives such as changing job or not driving to work. However, a lot of stress is actually how you perceive things internally. Do you let things get to you, or do you let things go? This is something that can change your relationship with stress significantly. For those who are not able to do this themselves, consider contacting a cognitive behavioural therapist.

+ Set aside 15 minutes every day for yourself to think, dream and not be pressurised by anything within your daily plans. Note: watching television is not relaxing as it is designed to keep you alert and awake.

+ Avoid a diet that puts further stress on your adrenals. This includes limiting alcohol to seven units a week, stopping caffeine intake – this puts quite a strain on the adrenals – and all diet and soft drink intake.

+ Stop consuming all fast-releasing sugars as they create a state of stress in the body, stimulating the release of cortisol. This means avoiding white bread and pasta, sweets, breakfast cereals, and anything else that has added sugar to it. Substitute these with complex carbohydrates that help to stabilise blood sugar levels, e.g. brown rice, wholemeal bread and pasta, oats and quinoa.

+ Avoid processed foods, food products that contain chemical additives, and all fried foods as these put an additional stress on the body.

+ Eat a well-balanced diet with lots of fruit and vegetables. If you are in a stressed state, you may need extra protein so go for protein-rich foods such as oily fish and eggs (or vegetable proteins if you don't eat animal products).

+ Avoid eating under stressful conditions. If you eat too quickly or under stress, you will not absorb your nutrients and your digestive system will not work well. Eat in a relaxed environment to ensure there is sufficient blood flow and effective digestion.

+ Exercise three times a week for 20 to 30 minutes – it's great for reducing anxiety and nervousness and for elevating your brain chemicals to make you feel good.

 # Supplements for stress

+ Magnesium
+ B vitamins
+ Vitamin C and bioflavonoids
+ Zinc
+ 'Adaptogenic' herbs, e.g. ashwaganda, astragalus, cordyceps, ginseng, rhodiola. These strengthen and improve the body's overall ability to cope with the affects of stress.

Hypoglycaemia

If you suffer periods during the day when you feel dizzy, irritable, become irrational – particularly when you haven't eaten for a few hours – then your blood sugar levels may be unbalanced.

Keeping your blood sugar balanced is very important, particularly for the brain, which uses 60 per cent of all the glucose in the body. It is also very important in helping you to lose weight, and, in many people, to stop them gaining weight. If you have a problem with weight loss then you probably have a marked blood sugar balancing problem – so read on.

This important balancing process is co-ordinated by a number of different hormones. When the pancreas registers high levels of glucose in the blood, often just after eating, it responds by releasing insulin. This makes the cells in the body take up glucose, which lowers blood levels and also stimulates the liver to store glucose as glycogen. On the other hand, if there is a shortage of glucose, say after exercise or when there is a long gap between meals, the pancreas will release another hormone to stimulate the liver to release more glucose.

Rapidly falling blood sugar levels, as when you're frightened, angry or stressed, will cause the release of stress hormones, adrenalin and cortisol from the adrenal glands. These cause a faster breakdown of stored glucose to provide extra energy for the perceived crisis. These hormones have other effects on the body causing anxiety and panic. This is why one of the major treatments for panic attacks is balancing blood sugar.

Frequently asked questions

Why does eating sugar and refined carbohydrates cause blood sugar problems?
When you eat 'fast' or refined sugars or carbohydrates found in cakes, biscuits, white bread, pasta and rice, these sugars rapidly enter the bloodstream and may cause a surge in glucose levels. The body releases insulin, lowering blood sugar levels. Too much insulin release – which can happen, particularly if the body is not very sensitive to insulin – will lead to the sugar being stored as fat and an overcorrection of the blood sugar level, causing you to feel hungry an hour later. And you will have now entered the fast sugar/insulin vicious circle.

Do complex carbohydrates and protein have the same effect?
Complex carbohydrates such as brown rice, bread and pasta are slowly broken down by the liver into glucose. This is then slowly released into the bloodstream at an even rate so you don't suffer the highs and lows. Similarly protein digestion is a slow process leading to steady glucose levels in the body.

Balancing the blood sugar is a finely tuned process but one that is constantly stressed in modern society by lifestyle and diet. As a result, hypoglycaemia, or a tendency to a low blood sugar, is increasingly common. Undesirable in itself, it's also a forerunner to diabetes, so you should take immediate steps to avoid risk factors (see below). Typical symptoms of hypoglycaemia are:

- Dizziness/light-headedness
- Mood swings
- Anxiety
- Irritability
- Aggressiveness

- Poor memory & concentration
- Difficulty making decisions
- Food cravings
- Blurred vision

- Seizure
- Heart palpitations
- Sweating
- Nervous stomach
- Frequent urination
- Insomnia

You can check your symptoms from the list above. Also, as a rough guide, if you develop symptoms three to four hours after eating and they disappear with eating, hypoglycaemia may well be your problem. Try following the Eating for Life food programme (see page 166) for one month; if your symptoms settle, then you have the diagnosis.

Medical tests can be arranged by your doctor to confirm diagnosis, but these can be time-consuming and, in the end, the treatment is still the same: i.e. maintaining a lifestyle and diet that balance your blood sugar better.

Hypoglycaemia risk factors

- Regularly eating sugary foods or refined carbohydrates.
- Regularly eating junk food, fast food or processed foods.
- Regularly drinking alcohol – alcohol causes a lowering of blood sugar levels.
- Smoking – acts like caffeine to upset blood sugar balance.
- Caffeine – drinking even moderate amounts of coffee, soft drinks, tea, medications and anything else containing caffeine has a very powerful and immediate effect of raising blood sugar levels. You may immediately feel better after a cup of coffee, and for an hour or two, but your falsely elevated blood sugar levels will soon fall again.
- High stress levels – causing more cortisol and adrenalin to be released.
- Not eating enough complex carbohydrate.
- Lack of protein in the diet and poor protein digestion.
- Excess exercise, which stresses the body.
- Adrenal fatigue.

Metabolic syndrome

If you are overweight and inactive then you may be setting the stage for a medical condition called metabolic syndrome or syndrome X.

It's a condition that most people don't know they have because there are very few symptoms in the early and middle stages. Yet it's a disorder that is becoming increasingly common, now affecting one in five Americans and 40 per cent of people in their sixties and seventies.

It is a condition that is caused by the body's inability to utilise insulin in the body properly – the so-called insulin resistance that you see in the pre-diabetic stage. Active muscle cells cannot take up glucose as easily as they should and so blood insulin levels are chronically higher, which inhibits our fat cells from giving up their energy stores to let us lose weight. It is therefore associated with obesity, hypertension, glucose intolerance and subsequently type-2 diabetes. There is a genetic influence for the condition but by far the most important predisposing factors are:

+ Increased weight – particularly with waist over 102cm (40in) in a man or 88cm (35in) in a woman

+ Diet high in refined carbohydrates

+ Lack of physical activity

+ Smoking

+ Post menopause

If you suspect that you may have metabolic syndrome, you should see your doctor for further examination and tests. It would also be beneficial to follow the action plan for type-2 diabetes overleaf.

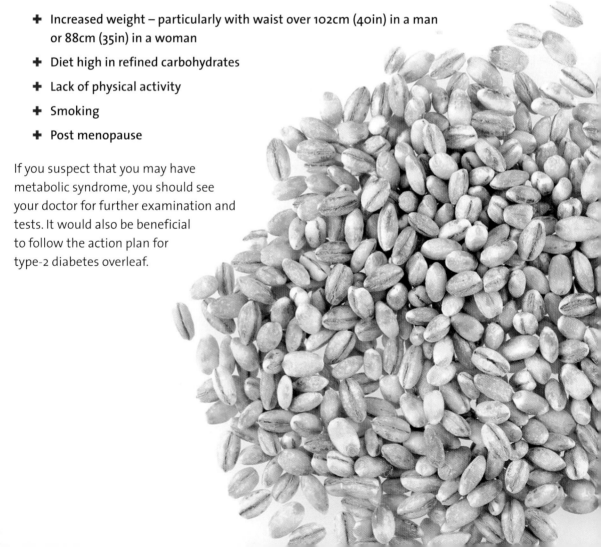

Type-2 diabetes

As many as 1.5 million people in Britain have been diagnosed with type-2 diabetes and there are probably a further million undiagnosed. Every year the figures for this serious, chronic disorder get worse. And why? The answer is clear: poor diets, lack of exercise, and obesity.

It's type-2 that gets most of the attention – type-1 diabetes is a very different disorder, where a lack of insulin raises the blood glucose levels. This condition commonly becomes apparent in childhood and, unlike type-2, is not related to obesity. People with type-2 diabetes, as well as being overweight, have a lack of sensitivity to insulin, which raises both insulin and glucose in the blood. They also tend to develop the condition later in life, which is why it's also called mature onset diabetes. Another name for it is diabetes mellitus, which literally means 'honey running through' and refers to the large amounts of sweet, glucose-filled urine excreted by someone with the condition.

Catch it while you can!

Type-2 diabetes doesn't strike overnight. For most people it develops gradually, taking as long as seven years to reach the full-blown condition. So there's time for you to nip it in the bud – if you wait until you actually have diabetes, you'll be at the lower end of the slippery slope.

The so-called pre-diabetic phase usually starts with excess weight and associated insulin resistance, which makes the pancreas secrete more and more insulin to control blood sugar levels. This is unfortunate for two reasons: first, the high insulin levels cause the body to convert more glucose into fat, leading to more weight gain; secondly, as the weight increases so does the insulin, so you are now in a vicious circle. You'll probably be experiencing dizziness, lethargy, irritability, sweating, headaches and even lack of co-ordination. In fully fledged diabetes, the glucose levels will be persistently high – so before things get that far, take steps to remedy the situation.

By following the Eating for Life food programme (see page 166), losing weight and doing regular exercise, you can turn this situation around. Your body will become much more sensitised to insulin as a result and you may find you lose even more weight. Supplements can help, too:

+ Chromium to help balance blood sugar
+ Glutamine to help with sugar cravings
+ Zinc citrate, picolinate or true food zinc which helps to produce insulin

As a good diet is so important with this, we recommend you consult with a good nutritionist.

Dealing with diabetes

When your blood glucose can no longer be controlled by insulin and is always at high levels, then you have type-2 diabetes. This serious condition can lead to long-term complications such as vision problems, kidney disease, ischaemic heart disease, stroke, high blood pressure, and poor circulation – particularly in the small arteries. This is why, in time, 50 per cent of men with diabetes become impotent and why there are more infections and ulcers in the feet of diabetics. Other symptoms include:

+ Increased thirst

+ Increased hunger

+ Dry mouth

+ Numbness or tingling in the feet and the hands

+ Nausea and occasional vomiting

+ Frequent urination

+ Blurred vision

+ Frequent infections of skin, urinary tract and vagina

 # Type-2 diabetes action plan

Aggressive control of blood sugar is critical to prevent complications. You also need to monitor your blood pressure very carefully, and keep it below 140/80 (see page 52). Having diabetes and high blood pressure considerably increases your risk of developing ischaemic heart disease.

+ Eat a diet high in complex carbohydrates – brown rice, brown bread and brown pasta.

+ Avoid sugar or sugar substitutes except honey (no more than 1 tablespoon per day).

+ Eat a low-fat diet. Avoid saturated fats as much as possible, including cheese, red meat and particularly junk or fast food.

+ Eat a high-fibre diet, including 6 to 8 helpings of vegetables and fruit per day.

+ Get your protein from chicken, fish, eggs and vegetable sources such as hummus, dhal, tofu and beans.

+ Eat lots of berries, grapes and plums. These contain phytochemicals that have a protective effect on the eye.

+ Take small meals frequently rather than big heavy meals hours apart. Eating less food at a time places less stress on the pancreas.

+ Keep alcohol consumption down to a moderate level, such as 7 units per week.

+ Reduce caffeine intake to no more than one cup of coffee per day.

+ Exercise helps to sensitise the tissues to insulin, control blood pressure and improve the lipid profile. Take aerobic exercise for half an hour, four times a week.

+ Drugs like metformin can be helpful at this stage, so work closely with your doctor on this.

✚ Monitoring type-2 diabetes

Checking your blood sugar levels is vital, so you should have a home glucose-monitoring machine. Initially, monitor your sugar levels several times a day so that you get a sense of how your own levels vary depending on your activity levels and diet.

Check your blood pressure and keep it below 140/80. See page 52.

Test your mineral levels, particularly zinc, magnesium and chromium which are often low. See page 39.

✎ Supplements for diabetes

People with diabetes have a tendency to lose high amounts of minerals in their urine, particularly zinc, which is very important for taste, and magnesium. Zinc deficiency causes blunted taste buds, which may explain sweet food cravings. Correcting this deficiency may be very important to prevent sugar cravings.

- ✚ A multivitamin or mineral formula
- ✚ Zinc
- ✚ Coenzyme Q10 to help protect the eyes
- ✚ Chromium to stabilise blood sugar
- ✚ Vitamin E to improve insulin activity

If you are taking warfarin you should consult with your doctor about vitamin E, and similarly if you are on diabetic medication and are considering taking chromium.

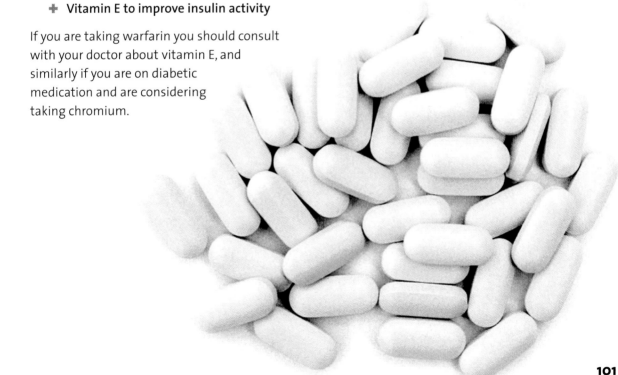

The brain
Your body's computer

It makes you think – that amazingly complex structure inside your head, with its intricate network of electric signals and chemical reactions. Weight for weight, no computer can challenge the capacity of the brain. It controls the myriad functions that keep you alive, and it has a strong influence on the person you are. Of all the organs in the body, the brain is the most sensitive to biochemical and nutritional deficiencies and imbalances. So your diet, through its effect on the production of brain chemicals, can influence your mood, behaviour, thought processes and emotional reactions. The more you know about the food/brain connection, the more empowered you are to make the dietary changes that benefit the brain – and your whole self.

Fat facts

Did you realise that 60 per cent of your brain is made up of fat – the right kinds of fat, that is. The right fats are essential for almost every aspect of the brain's structure and function.

There are four main kinds of fat, two of which can't be made in the body and so must be included in your diet. These are the fatty acids omega-3 (found in fish and flaxseed oil) and omega-6 (found in sunflower oil and oil of evening primrose.

The other two fats – docosahexaenoic acid (DHA) and arachidonic acid (AA) – can either be made in the body or consumed directly. However, the conversion of these fats in the body can be compromised by stress, infections, excess sugar, and lack of vitamins and minerals.

What you shouldn't have in your diet are trans fatty acids. These are formed when vegetable oils are 'hydrogenated', which stabilises them and lengthens their shelf life. Such oils are used in margarines and other spreads, in fact a huge range of packaged and pre-cooked foods, both savoury and sweet. Look on the label for 'partially hydrogenated oil' – and beware. Trans fatty acids can rob the body of the correct fatty acids and take their place in the brain's cells and nerves, which then become quite rigid and don't work properly. Result: impaired mental function.

Sweet reason

The most important nutrient for the brain and nervous system is glucose, with the brain using 60 per cent of the body's supply. However, it needs to be balanced carefully, within a narrow range. Too much glucose can damage nerve cells. On the other hand, give the brain too little glucose and you may experience dizziness, clouded vision, irritability, emotional instability, headaches, sweating and tremors.

Messages within the brain

Within that familiar image of an overgrown walnut is an enormous mass of interconnected nerve cells – around 100 billion of them. These communicate with each other at junctions through the release of chemical messengers called neurotransmitters. Brain function fundamentally depends on how the different parts communicate with each other, so good mental health depends on having good sending and receiving sites and optimum levels of neurotransmitters.

Don't go bananas!

Dr Wendy says: 'The husband of a friend of mine carries bananas with him when they're travelling together. When I asked him why, he said it's because she turns from being a lovely woman to a highly argumentative one in the space of a few minutes when her blood sugar drops. Having a quick fix at the ready has drastically reduced their marital spats. Sound familiar?'

Diet and neurotransmitters

Neurotransmitters are made from proteins consumed in food. If your diet is deficient in the building blocks then you will not be able to make these neurotransmitters, and mental and neurological disorders may result.

Dopamine

This neurotransmitter works like a natural amphetamine controlling your metabolism, energy, excitement about new ideas and motivation. It controls bodily functions such as blood pressure and digestion. It also generates the electricity that controls voluntary movement. When it is out of balance, you can get addictive disorders, obesity, severe fatigue and in the long run Parkinson's disease.

Dopamine is made from phenylalanine, found in beets, soybeans, almonds, eggs, meat and grains. It requires vitamin B12, folic acid and magnesium for its production.

Serotonin

When your levels of serotonin are balanced, you sleep well, enjoy food and think rationally. When the levels are out of balance, you may experience sleep problems, depression, hormone imbalances, PMS and eating disorders.

Serotonin is made from tryptophan, found in eggs, turkey, bananas, yogurt, milk, cottage cheese and dates. It requires vitamin B6 for its production and carbohydrates to be more readily absorbed.

Acetylcholine

A brain lubricant, acetylcholine keeps the internal structures of the body moist so that energy and information can pass easily around the system. When your levels are balanced you are creative and feel good about yourself. When they're out of balance you may get language disorders and memory loss.

Acetylcholine is made from choline, found in eggs, liver and soybeans.

GABA

Natural valium! It controls the brain's rhythm so you function at a steady rate both mentally and physically. When it is out of balance you can get headaches, palpitations, seizures, low libido, and heart problems.

GABA is made from glutamine, found in flour and potatoes.

The neurotransmitters

There are four primary neurotransmitters. Two of them are often bandied about in articles about diet and health: dopamine and serotonin. The other two are less well known to most people: acetylcholine and GABA (gamma-aminobutyric acid) .

When our bodies are in dynamic balance, then there is a free flow of these chemicals. If there is an excess, the junctions become flooded and signals can't wade through to the receptor terminal on the receiving nerve cell or neuron. On the other hand, if there is a deficiency the nerve signals have nothing on which to travel to the other side of the junction, so the message is never carried. Other parts of the body will react to these imbalances by either overworking or shutting down.

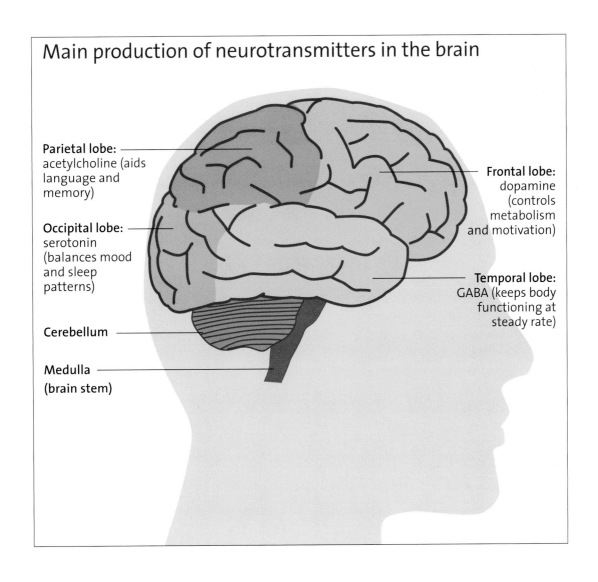

Main production of neurotransmitters in the brain

Parietal lobe: acetylcholine (aids language and memory)

Occipital lobe: serotonin (balances mood and sleep patterns)

Cerebellum

Medulla (brain stem)

Frontal lobe: dopamine (controls metabolism and motivation)

Temporal lobe: GABA (keeps body functioning at steady rate)

Improve your state of mind

Other factors influence brain chemicals. Exposure to natural light has a very beneficial effect. If you're not able to work or live in an environment with exposure to sunlight during the day, then you should get out in the middle of the day for 20 minutes to expose your eyes to natural sunlight, without wearing sunglasses. If you can't do this, then buy a light box that emits full-spectrum lighting, or fit special full-spectrum light bulbs. Turn these on for two hours in your house or office every day.

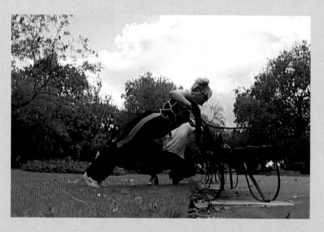

A quicker way to raise all levels of brain chemicals is, quite simply, exercise. Do it, ideally, in the open air in daylight for maximum benefit.

Hormone levels also have an effect. Low oestrogen, for instance, leads to low serotonin, which may be why women are more prone to depression in the menopause. Keeping stress levels down is very important, as raised cortisol and noradrenalin can make you angry, lose concentration, lower your potential for learning, decrease quality of sleep and increase mood swings.

As well as diet, light, exercise and hormones, being exposed to certain chemicals also influences our state of thinking, for good or ill. For instance, taking cocaine can make some people anxious and paranoid, whereas taking valerian, which acts on the brain's GABA receptor, provides a tranquillising effect, helping with sleeplessness, hysteria and anxiety. Finally, and perhaps most importantly, thinking positive thoughts can influence our brain chemistry.

However, while you can take steps to improve the way your brain works – and therefore your state of mind and your enjoyment of life – our moods do still fluctuate for a variety of reasons. Having a low mood is a natural phenomenon in most people's lives at some time. In some people this low mood becomes sustained over a longer period, and then they may be diagnosed as being depressed.

Exposure to natural light has a beneficial effect on the brain

Depression

Depression is a very common disorder, affecting some three million people in Britain every year – and rising. Women are three times more likely than men to suffer from it, perhaps because depression is related to low serotonin levels, and women make less serotonin than men. Typical features of depression are:

+ Low mood

+ Fatigue and lethargy

+ Decreased appetite or comfort-eating

+ Inability to make decisions

+ Insomnia

+ Lack of interest in sex

+ Crying all the time

+ Guilty feelings

+ Anxiety

If you have three or more of these features, your mood needs a boost. Six or more and you may well be depressed – consult a nutritionist and your doctor.

There are many causes of depression, which are beyond the scope of this book. What you do need to know is that while drugs can be useful – and some do indeed transform sufferers' lives – you can influence your own moods and brain chemicals by simply changing what you eat and the way you live.

 Quick tips

+ If you're depressed and menopausal, and don't want to take HRT (hormone replacment therapy), then try 5HTP (5-Hydroxitryptophan) to raise your serotonin levels (although usage should be avoided if you are on any other anti-depressant medication).

+ If you are on a weight-loss programme, then you too may benefit from taking 5HTP as it will control appetite and help balance blood sugar levels, as well as making your mood more positive (again, usage should be avoided if you are on any other anti-depressant medication).

+ If you're on the pill and are feeling depressed, then consider whether you want to continue taking this form of contraception as it frequently causes depression. If you do want to continue taking it, then try supplementing with B vitamins and zinc as these become depleted in conjunction with birth control pill use.

+ Try exercise. It aids the release of serotonin and recent studies have shown that it not only improves self-image but can be as effective as taking antidepressants.

Depression action plan

+ Keep up vitamin and mineral levels. Depression has been linked to deficiencies of B vitamins, zinc, magnesium and essential fatty acids. The B vitamins, zinc and magnesium are important in the production of serotonin, while the higher the levels of omega-3 fatty acids in the body, the higher the levels of serotonin.

+ Cut out junk food, fast food, processed and sugary foods – a common cause of depression. The body has to supply its own vital vitamins and minerals to process the chemicals and sugar as these foods don't bring their own.

+ Eat enough carbohydrates. A diet with no carbohydrates can make you depressed, as the body uses them to make serotonin – which is why when you're depressed you crave carbohydrates. Make sure you take complex carbohydrates, as blood sugar imbalances can be an important contributor to depression.

+ Avoid saturated fats. Not only do foods rich in saturated fat lower your levels of the essential fatty acids, omega-3 and 6, but they also slow down the blood flow to the brain as the blood cells become more sticky and tend to clump together – this leads to sluggishness, slow thinking and fatigue.

+ Check for food sensitivities. Many people's brains are sensitive to certain foods, the commonest being wheat and dairy. Try cutting out one or both of these from your diet for a month and see how you feel. (See pages 179–183.)

+ Be careful with alcohol. Many people who are depressed drink to excess; in terms of lifestyle factors, it may be the commonest contributor to depression after faulty diets. When you drink, initially the increase in blood sugar feels great – the brain loves the sugar rush. However, after about an hour the true effects of alcohol start to set in. It's really a brain depressant, which is why it was used in the days before anaesthetics to calm patients who needed surgery. What is also not commonly realised is that for 24 hours after drinking you will feel more anxious than normal, which is why most people are grabbing a drink the next day. So not only depression but also anxiety sets in. Alcohol also depletes the body of essential fatty acids and B vitamins crucial for neurotransmitter production.

+ Avoid using recreational drugs. Most of these are stimulants which, like alcohol, may make you feel great while you're taking them – but you crash later. What goes up must come down!

+ Stop smoking. Smokers are more likely to be depressed than non-smokers, due to the effects on circulation in the brain and also the lowering of vital minerals such as vitamin C and zinc.

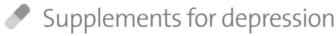 Supplements for depression

+ Good multivitamin and mineral, with plenty of B vitamins, particularly B6.

+ Omega-3 fish oils.

+ Magnesium, especially in the evening.

+ Calcium (if you're not eating dairy).

+ Zinc picolinate or true food zinc (as well as the multivitamin).

+ 5 HTP-serotone. This needs to be taken with some carbohydrate at night to be well absorbed, e.g. a banana or a couple of wholewheat crackers. It is particularly effective if you are having problems sleeping but may need to be prescribed by a doctor. It should be avoided if you are on any other anti-depressant medication.

+ St John's wort is great for combating depression (in Germany, it's used much more commonly than in the UK – up to 50 per cent of patients are treated in this way). It has been shown to be just as effective as prescribed drugs for mild to moderate depression, but not for severe depression. (It may make the birth control pill less effective, so you may need a higher dose of pill or to change your form of contraception).

If none of this helps, then you may need professional help. Your doctor may diagnose underlying conditions contributing to depression, such as an underactive thyroid or vitamin B12 deficiency, or may change the medication that is contributing to your depression.

Drugs and diets apart, another really important factor for good mental – and physical – health is just what you can't manage when you're depressed: a good night's sleep.

Sleep

A good sleep is essential for rebuilding the body. The golden hours are between 11pm and 3am, but most people require seven to eight hours per night. During the night, growth hormone is released and this triggers proteins throughout the body to build new cells and repair any damage. It also allows the brain to resynchronise the brain's functions so that you wake re-energised the next day.

Most of us will have the occasional night when we don't sleep well. In fact, in a year, a third of the population will experience insomnia. If this is a regular occurrence, it will leave you feeling tired and irritable while experiencing blood sugar highs and lows, and poor quality memory and concentration.

Sleeping problems are usually caused by a serotonin imbalance, although sometimes GABA imbalances can cause problems as well. By building up your serotonin, not only will you sleep better, but your dopamine and acetylcholine will be replenished.

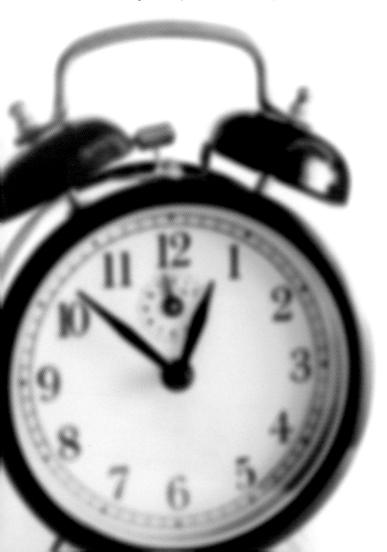

Eating too much of the wrong sort of food, too late in the evening, leads to sleepless nights

Sleep action plan

- Try to wind down. You need to have a routine of relaxation before going to bed such as a hot bath, so that the stress hormones produced by activity are allowed to decrease. At the same time the body starts to pump out serotonin and other brain chemicals that initiate sleep.

- Reduce your caffeine intake. This can be one of the fastest ways to improve your sleep. Ideally, drink no coffee after midday and no tea after 5pm. Limit your caffeine intake from chocolate as well, and eliminate soft drinks from your diet as almost all of these contain caffeine. If you have a serious sleeping problem, you may need to eliminate caffeine altogether.

- Reduce your alcohol intake. Most people know that if they drink too much alcohol they'll fall into a stupor – hardly a true sleep. But even in small quantities, alcohol can impair sleep in a number of ways. First, it releases adrenalin, a stimulating hormone designed to prepare the body for fight or flight. Second, it impairs the transport of tryptophan into the brain – an important precursor of serotonin. Third, it may adversely affect blood sugar balance (see page 136).

- Take exercise. Regular exercise also promotes good sleep, but make sure you finish your exercise at least three hours before bedtime.

- Eat earlier (and less) in the evening. Many people now eat their main meal of the day late in the evening. The problem is that by this time our digestive system starts to shut down and is relatively sluggish compared to earlier in the day. We then aggravate the situation by eating foods like cheese, red meat and saturated fatty foods such as chips, which require a considerable amount of time and energy to digest. So in order to get a better night's sleep, eat a lighter evening meal and finish eating before 8pm. You can also aid digestion and promote relaxation by drinking peppermint or camomile herbal teas.

- Balance your hormones. Women in the menopause have low oestrogen levels, which tend to cause low serotonin levels. Balancing the hormones can be very helpful, as can antidepressant drugs that raise serotonin levels. However, if this applies to you, first try diet, exercise, reducing alcohol, and taking B6, zinc, magnesium and essential fats, as these help menopausal symptoms and raise serotonin levels.

- Get your minerals right. Many of us are deficient in minerals, so checking your intake of calcium and, especially, magnesium – two very important minerals for sleeping – could be very helpful (see page 39). To increase intake of these minerals in your diet, see the section on foods containing calcium and magnesium (pages 141–2). However, a quick way to increase your calcium is to drink a cup of hot milk before bed. To boost magnesium, try eating more wholegrains, broccoli and cauliflower at dinner, or take a supplement in the evening.

the brain

There's something else that can disturb your sleep, sometimes severely, but for once it's nothing to do with you – it's when you're within earshot of a heavy snorer.

Snoring

Millions of people snore, with men being more likely to do so than women. Snoring is caused by the vibration of the uvula – the cone-shaped piece of flesh that drops down from the soft palate at the back of the roof of the mouth – during sleep. The deeper the sleep, the more the palate muscles relax. So, depending on the person's anatomy, during deep sleep the soft palate muscles may relax to such an extent that the uvula vibrates during normal breathing, causing snoring. The chances of snoring are much greater if the nose or nasal passage is blocked because then the person breathes through their open mouth. Obstruction can be due to nasal polyps, congestion, a deviated nasal septum, enlarged tonsils, adenoids or loose dentures.

Also, most people who snore do so when they are lying on their backs, because this causes the jaw to drop open and the tongue to fall backwards, causing more vibration of the uvula and partial closing of the windpipe.

 # Snoring action plan

+ Lose weight – obesity increases the risk of snoring threefold because fat settles around the soft palate and its muscles, and weight will alter the action of the palate.

+ Reduce salt intake – too much salt leads to fluid retention.

+ Indigestion can make snoring worse, so avoid it by finishing meals at least two hours before bedtime (you may also benefit from taking a digestive enzyme).

+ Reduce alcohol intake and stop drinking at least two hours before bedtime.

+ Sleep on your side, not on your back.

+ Try elevating your head by adding an extra pillow.

+ Stop over-the-counter antihistamines/tranquilisers (don't stop prescribed medication without consulting your doctor first).

+ Stop smoking.

If all these home remedies fail, then you should consult your doctor, who will see if there is any underlying cause. Often a steroid nasal spray is enough. There are also mechanical devices that can resolve the problem. Otherwise, it is probably worth having a sleep study arranged, to monitor pulse, brainwaves, breathing and oxygen levels during sleep. This will help diagnose if there is a more serious problem such as obstructive sleep apnoea.

Obesity increases the risk of snoring three-fold

Sleep apnoea

Have you ever slept with a snorer who suddenly stops breathing – and you wonder if they're ever going to take a breath again? You lie there willing the person to breathe and, just as you're about to call 999, they gag, gasp and then start to breathe normally again. Someone who does this may have sleep apnoea.

This is a serious problem, often associated with snoring. A sufferer has very irregular breathing, which may cause repeated waking. What it certainly causes are periods when the person stops breathing for anything from ten seconds to two minutes. When the breathing stops, the level of oxygen in the blood drops, resulting in oxygen deprivation to the brain. The build-up of carbon dioxide in the blood prompts the person to gag and gasp and start breathing again. This cycle may go on up to 200 times per night. The person doesn't get a good refreshing sleep and so feels exhausted and drowsy the next day. (And any sleeping partner – who's been kept awake and on tenterhooks – won't feel too good either.)

Because the sleep is non-restorative and involves oxygen deprivation in the brain, a number of health disorders are commonly associated with this: increased blood pressure, and an increased risk of heart disease and strokes. People with sleep apnoea also tend to have extreme sleepiness during the day, which makes working and driving hazardous. They have a higher than average incidence of driving accidents and emotional disorders, and are much more likely to have concentration and memory problems.

Sleep apnoea treatment

Dr Wendy says: 'The treatment is much the same as for snoring. However, because the condition is potentially much more serious, I would recommend that you give up alcohol and sedative drugs of any kind, and lose weight as soon as possible. If these simple measures don't work for you, then you may have to use a special "CPAP" machine, which continuously pumps air into the airway via a mask to keep it open during sleep. This, while effective, is not without its drawbacks. As ever, it's worth making changes in your diet and lifestyle to have a better chance of avoiding such extreme remedies.'

The skin
On the surface

Making a good impression is crucial, and one of the first things that people notice is the quality of your skin. Looking healthy begins with having good skin.

Not only is the skin the outer covering of the skeleton and internal organs but, directly or indirectly, it is linked to almost every organ in the body. Furthermore, in its own right it is the body's largest organ, weighing up to 16 per cent of the body's total weight. It is unique to each individual, each race and even different parts of the same body. Despite this, all skin has the same basic structure.

Getting under the skin

What you see is only the top layer, the epidermis, which contains the pigment or melanin that gives the skin its colour. This layer protects the skin, acting as a resistant surface that is constantly being replaced every three weeks or so as dead cells are rubbed away. The middle layer is the dermis – the most vital part of the skin, linking it to the rest of the body with nerves, blood vessels, sweat glands and hair follicles; while the skin's oil glands lubricate it, elastin gives it tone and makes it supple, and collagen gives it strength and structure. The third, subcutaneous, layer is a storage depot for fat. This provides a protective padding but also gives the skin a full, healthy look.

What the skin does

While we can't fail to notice that the skin protects our insides from the outside world, it has many other functions, some of which are more familiar than others.

✚ Heat regulation

Skin produces sweat when we're too hot and goose bumps when we're cold (the little hairs stand up to give insulation).

✚ Absorption

It's a great surface to absorb drugs/creams. (There's a longstanding belief – thankfully changing – that something put on the skin won't be absorbed into the body. Don't kid yourself!)

✚ Excretion

The skin is an important organ of detoxification, assisting the colon, lungs and kidneys in eliminating waste through skin oils and sweat.

✚ Resistance to bacterial attack

As the cells of the top layer of skin are constantly being rubbed off, this also dislodges harmful bacteria – so the skin is an important part of the immune system.

✚ Sense of touch

The skin has an amazing amount of nerve endings and is constantly feeding back information to the brain.

✚ Synthesis of vitamin D and melanin

Vitamin D is used by every cell in the body and is very important for our immunity and bone building. Melanin gives us our suntans.

The skin is the body's most visible organ of elimination so spots or rashes can be a sign of imbalance in the body

the skin

Being so large and so visible, any change in the skin tends to be noticeable – it's open to all kinds of rashes, spots and other eruptions, which may indicate a specific skin disorder, or be related to disease elsewhere in the body. In either case, research has shown that eliminating dairy and gluten from the diet may be beneficial in any skin condition.

Bruising

Most of the time when you bruise yourself, you're not even aware of what injury it was that caused the blood vessels in the subcutaneous layer of the skin to leak and release blood. Many women notice that they bruise more easily around the time of their period. This is due to a change in hormones in the body at this time, and may be aggravated by using aspirin, ibuprofen and other non-steroidal anti-inflammatory drugs which always tend to make you bruise more.

Other factors that lead to increased bruising are blood-thinning drugs, vitamin E supplementation, lack of vitamin C and bioflavonoids in the diet, and a poor digestive system.

 ## Bruising action plan

+ Stop using aspirin and non-steroidal anti-inflammatories (if possible).
+ Eat a diet rich in vitamin C and bioflavonoids such as kiwi fruit, citrus fruits, berries and cabbage.
+ Chew your food well.
+ Improve your digestion (see pages 60–83).

 ## Supplements for bruising

+ Vitamin C.
+ Good multivitamin and mineral containing bioflavonoids such as grape seed extract, lutein and bilberry.
+ Limit vitamin E usage.
+ Digestive enzymes with each meal to improve your digestion (if needed).

    If all of this fails, then see your doctor. Rarely, bruising can be due to a severe underlying medical condition.

Acne

Many of us had spots as a teenager and felt very self-conscious about them – and it can be disconcerting to continue having them into adult life.

Acne breaks out when the sebaceous glands produce too much sebum and keratin, blocking the skin pores and making them more likely to get infected. Exactly why this happens is not entirely understood, but acne is an inflammatory skin disorder related to hormones and detoxification.

Acne is much more common in overweight people as they tend to sweat more easily to reduce heat and have more need to detoxify through the skin. The toxic waste irritates the skin and sets the stage for acne and other skin conditions. So if the functioning of the liver (the body's most important organ of detoxification), is improved, then acne is often improved.

 ## Acne action plan

+ Avoid fried foods and those high in saturated fats, e.g. junk food and convenience food, as these make the skin pores more likely to get blocked.

+ Do what all fashion models do and drink 8 glasses of water a day to help the kidneys flush out the toxins in the urine.

+ Avoid sugar as it promotes bacterial growth on the skin.

+ Eat plenty of zinc-rich food, which is good for any skin condition, e.g. shellfish, turkey and brown rice.

+ Eat sulphur-rich food, also good for the skin, e.g. eggs, onions and garlic.

+ Stop smoking – it increases toxins in the body and also depletes vitamin C and zinc, both of which are important for skin health.

 ## Supplements for acne

+ Multivitamin and mineral supplement
+ Zinc picolinate
+ MSM
+ Acidophilus
+ Vitamin C, especially if you smoke

If these simple remedies don't do the trick, consider consulting a nutritionist or an expert in Chinese herbal medicine and acupuncture – these can have excellent results – or see your doctor with a view to medication.

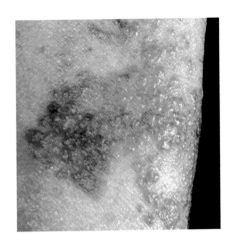

Dermatitis

Dermatitis is an inflammation of the skin that produces scaling, flaking, itching, thickening and colour changes. Many cases of dermatitis are due to some form of allergy resulting from contact with a range of substances from metals to perfumes. It can also be due to sensitivity to specific foods or sunlight, a reaction to drugs, or stress, particularly chronic anxiety. Sometimes it can be caused by a combination of these factors working together, which is why people will say, 'I never used to be sensitive to that.'

It is much more common in overweight people, whose levels of inflammatory chemicals are much higher in the body and in whom the skin tends to be used more as an organ for eliminating waste. Both of these factors irritate the skin.

 ## Dermatitis action plan

+ Aim for a diet low in red meat and saturated fats.

+ Avoid dairy and wheat products altogether for one month and see if there is an improvement.

+ Remove citrus fruits from the diet as these may aggravate the skin.

+ Follow a diet high in omega-3 oils such as fish and seeds.

+ Eat at least 6 to 8 helpings of vegetables and fruit a day.

+ Get tested for food and contact allergies, and avoid the indicated foods.

 ## Supplements for dermatitis

+ Omega-3 fish oils
+ Vitamin E
+ Evening oil of primrose (take with evening meal)
+ Vitamin C
+ Multivitamin and mineral with bilberry and lutein

Urticaria or hives

This is an inflammatory condition that appears suddenly as red, itchy welts on the skin. It's brought on by an allergy to something, and this allergy causes a release of histamine into the skin which produces the itching, swelling and redness. The allergies may be due to:

+ Drugs – particularly antibiotics and anti-inflammatories
+ Chemicals put on the skin
+ Chemicals used in the house or workplace
+ Food – commonly nuts, berries, shellfish and, more recently, in meat products because of the widespread use of antibiotics in animal feed

Urticaria action plan

The most obvious course of action in treating hives is to identify the thing that caused it, and avoid it. Unfortunately, this can often prove to be very difficult. The first-line treatment of hives is antihistamines, which can be bought over the counter or prescribed by your doctor. However, in a chronic situation you are much better off trying a change in diet and lifestyle, as antihistamines are suppressive agents and may actually make hives worse.

+ Avoid all nuts, berries, shellfish and citrus fruits.
+ Eat foods that are not pro-inflammatory (see page 123).
+ Avoid white wine as its additives may aggravate the condition.

Supplements for urticaria

+ Aloe vera gel applied to the affected skin
+ Acidophilus to replace good gut bacteria
+ Vitamin C to lower histamine levels
+ Quercetin to reduce inflammation
+ Calcium to help lower histamine levels

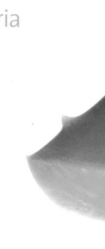

the skin

Rosacea

Rosacea is a chronic inflammatory skin disorder with patchy flushing and/or acne eruption around the cheeks, nose and forehead. It's a very common condition, affecting 10 per cent of people in the UK, particularly those who are overweight. It usually appears after the age of 30 and affects three times more women than men. The men who are affected tend to get it much more severely, often producing that characteristic 'Father Christmas' nose (red and enlarged). The tendency can be inherited, but most commonly it is associated with diet and lifestyle. Changes here can bring great improvements.

 ## Rosacea action plan

- Avoid all fast food, junk food and pre-packaged food.
- Avoid spicy food and citrus fruits.
- Reduce alcohol.
- Avoid coffee.
- Avoid constipation – rosacea is affected by bowel habits.
- Don't use skin products containing alcohol.
- Reduce stress.
- Avoid extremes of temperature.
- Get tested for food intolerances(see page 69) and contact allergies.

 ## Supplements for rosacea

- Vitamin B complex
- Zinc, preferably food state or picolinate
- Good multivitamin and mineral to guard against common deficiencies
- Acidophilus to build good bowel bacteria
- Milk thistle to help the liver detoxify the blood
- Oil of evening primrose

Do not use steroid creams. These thin the skin in the longterm and do not get rid of the underlying problem – when you stop using them, the problem will recur and often be worse. In most cases consultation with a nutritionist or a specialist in traditional Chinese medicine can be helpful.

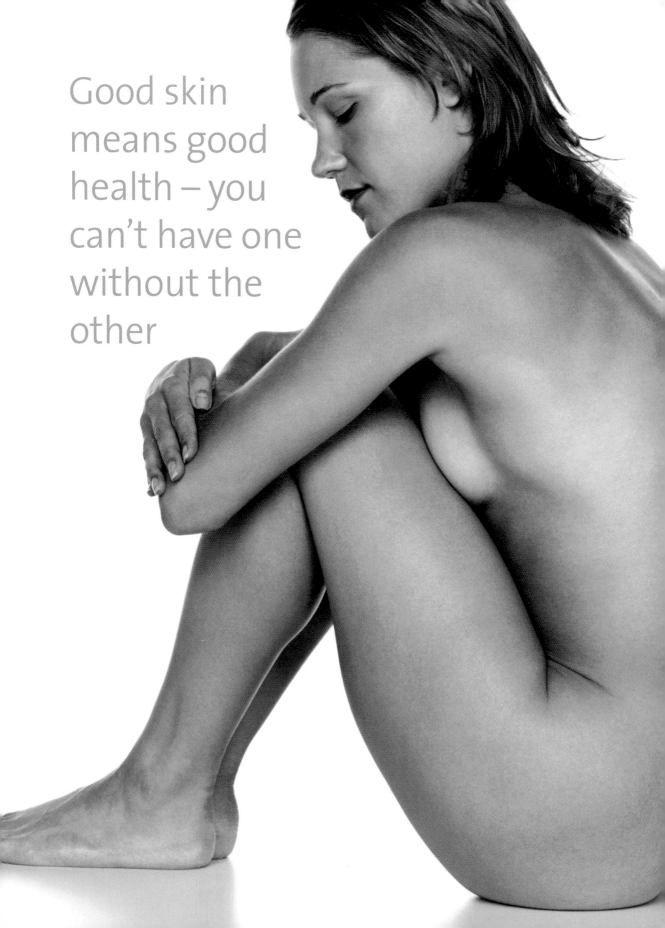

Good skin means good health – you can't have one without the other

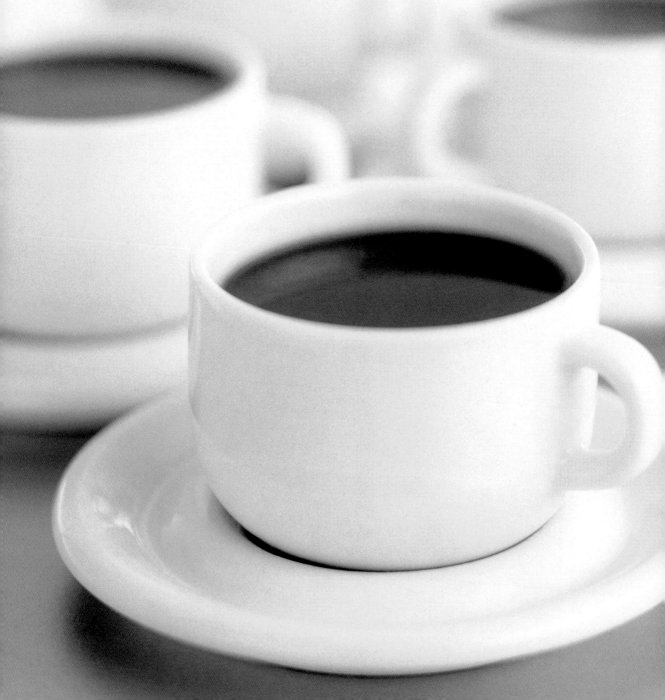

Avoid all drinks containing caffeine to help combat inflammatory conditions

Anti-inflammatory diet

This diet is beneficial for inflammatory conditions including the skin conditions rosacea, dermatitis and urticaria as well as rheumatoid arthritis and gout.

Eat less...

+ Saturated fats in your diet – so avoid red meat, dairy, deep-fried foods, takeaway and ready-made meals.

+ Coffee and soft drinks containing caffeine.

+ Citrus fruits.

+ Spicy food – particularly paprika.

+ Sugar and all foods containing sugar.

+ Alcohol – a maximum of one glass of red wine per day. The red skins are high in bioflavonoids which are powerful antioxidants.

Eat more...

+ Extra virgin olive oil instead of vegetable oils. It is high in anti-inflammatory omega-9 fatty acids.

+ Omega-3 fatty acids – eat more salmon, sardines, mackerel, sea bass, or flaxseed oil if you are a vegetarian.

+ Vitamin C found in kiwis, beetroot, green leafy vegetables and sweet potatoes. This lowers anti-inflammatory chemicals as well as being important for collagen, cartilage and bone remodelling.

+ Fresh pineapple – it contains bromelain which is a natural anti-inflammatory.

+ Ginger – it contains over 500 compounds many of which are anti-inflammatory in nature.

+ Vitamin E found in nuts, seeds, eggs and brown rice. Working with vitamin C, it is a strong antioxidant and also improves the healing of tissues.

+ Garlic.

+ Green tea.

+ Berries – they are good antioxidants.

+ Foods containing sulphur such as eggs, asparagus, garlic and onions.

The joints
Getting connected

The skeleton key to health? Strong bones and supple joints allow you to move freely and energetically. There's nothing so aging as creaking knees and dodgy hips, and very little so painful. If you're overweight, you'll be making things worse by putting an immense strain on all the bones, muscles, joints and ligaments that have to support those extra pounds. And you're more likely to develop arthritis as a result, with your joints inflamed and literally wearing away. So if you're not as active as you were, and you feel your joints are getting stiff, now's the time to nip those twinges in the bud.

Joint account

Wherever two bones meet, there's a joint. The main joints in the body are synovial joints, which, with a tiny fluid-filled gap between them, allow free movement in many directions. This fluid is the body's very own brake oil: synovial fluid, which reduces friction between bones and absorbs shock. Where the bone surfaces meet at a joint, they are covered with cartilage, a firm but flexible tissue, which plays a similar role – providing a smooth and resilient surface that eases movement and cushions impact. It has no blood supply of its own and relies on the synovial fluid to supply it with oxygen and nutrients and to remove carbon dioxide and waste.

The synovial joint is surrounded by a capsule composed of two layers: the inner synovial membrane and the outer fibrous layer that holds the joint together, along with the muscles and ligaments. When these joints become inflamed, it is the synovial membrane that is affected initially, causing the all-too-common arthritis (which simply means 'joint inflammation'). The two main types of arthritis are osteoarthritis and the inflammatory conditions which include rheumatoid arthritis and gout.

A typical synovial joint

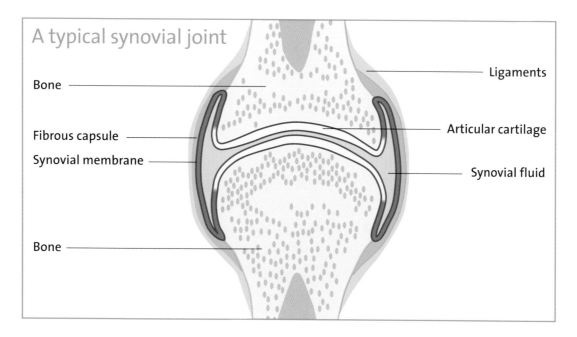

Bone

Fibrous capsule

Synovial membrane

Bone

Ligaments

Articular cartilage

Synovial fluid

The bare bones

If you think of bones what do you see? White, lifeless, solid, skeleton parts? They may be whitish but, beneath the surface, bones are hotbeds of teeming life: complex networks of blood vessels, nerves and cell production. What's more, they aren't solid – they're more like a honeycomb, made up of a mixture of hard minerals (calcium is the best known) and flexible collagen (a protein). Bones have a fantastic capacity to renew themselves and do so throughout your life – in fact, by the time you die, they'll be a lot younger than you!

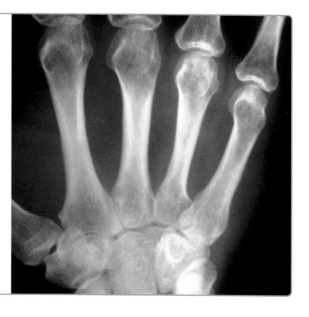

the joints

Osteoarthritis

Osteoarthritis ('osteo' meaning bone) is the 'wear and tear' arthritis, affecting up to 80 per cent of the population. The cartilage gets worn down and the synovial fluid dries up causing damage to the bony joint surfaces through lack of cushioning (leading to wear and tear). The ligaments around the joint shorten, limiting flexibility. The spine, knees, hips and any previously damaged joint are the most commonly affected. It runs in families, starting usually in middle age (or younger if you are overweight) and affects more women than men.

Progressing gradually, the commonest symptoms are pain and stiffness. The pain tends to get worse as the day progresses, and the stiffness is aggravated by activity. Initially, there is little inflammation, and the joint movement is limited by pain and muscle spasm. Later, inflammation becomes a much bigger problem, causing less flexibility and painful movement.

 ## Osteoarthritis action plan

+ Avoid undue stress and strain to the joints.
+ If your job involves heavy labour, change to a less physically demanding one.
+ Lose weight.
+ Don't smoke.
+ Avoid sugar, citrus fruits, red meat, cheese, coffee and excess alcohol.
+ Eat more green leafy vegetables, vegetable proteins, oily fish, onions and kelp. Aim for at least 8 helpings of fruit and vegetables per day.
+ Try stretching, walking and swimming to strengthen the muscles and maintain flexibility.

 ## Supplements for osteoarthritis

+ Glucosamine sulphate
+ Chondroitin sulphate
+ Fish oils
+ Calcium, unless you are eating a lot of dairy foods
+ Magnesium
+ Vitamin D
+ MSM – if inflamed

You may find that acupuncture helps, while over-the-counter anti-inflammatory drugs can ease the pain in the short term but should be avoided as much as possible in the long term because of side effects on the body. Your doctor should be consulted if these simple measures don't help.

Rheumatoid arthritis

Rheumatoid arthritis is an auto-immune condition caused by the immune system mistakenly attacking the body's own tissues, particularly the synovial fluid lining the joints. The joints most affected are the hands, wrists, feet, ankles and knees symmetrically on both sides of the body and usually in more than one joint. The inflammation causes the symptoms which are pain, stiffness and swelling. The stiffness tends to be worse first thing in the morning and gets better as the day progresses.

The inflamed synovial membrane sends out enzymes that break down the cartilage of the joint. Later this is replaced by fibrous tissue that calcifies and knots bones together, possibly restricting joint function. It is this process that causes the long-term problems in this condition. Rheumatoid arthritis usually occurs in the 20–40 age group but it can affect any age. It is more common in those who are obese, probably because it is an inflammatory condition. In 20 per cent of sufferers it will burn itself out, whereas in others it remains for life. It can be associated with inflammation under the skin, the heart and eyes.

Unfortunately many people with this condition will require medication from their doctor but, by following an anti-inflammatory diet (see page 123) and taking appropriate supplements, it can be helped.

 ## Supplements for rheumatoid arthritis

- ✚ Fish oils in high doses
- ✚ Flaxseed oil
- ✚ Multivitamin and mineral supplement containing bioflavonoid
- ✚ Bromelain
- ✚ MSM

Weight and arthritis

Overweight people are more likely to suffer from arthritis – but why? The key is inflammation. Overweight people tend to be in what's called a pro-inflammatory state, which is when the body's immune system is overstimulated and releases excessive amounts of the chemicals associated with the inflammatory process. Not surprisingly, overweight people are then more susceptible to inflammatory conditions of the synovial joints such as rheumatoid arthritis (in which the body attacks itself), gout and the later stages of osteoarthritis.

Gout

Gout used to be considered a rich man's disease because only those who could afford plentiful meat, cheese and wine (usually port) were thought to be affected by this condition. It's now seen much more across the social spectrum, but most often in men between the ages of 40 and 50. It also tends to run in families. The real cause of this form of inflammatory arthritis is too much uric acid in the blood, which then forms crystal deposits in joints, tendons, cartilage and kidneys.

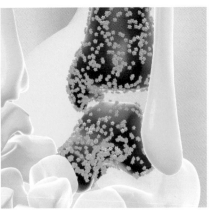

Gout usually attacks the joints of the feet, especially the big toe, but may also affect the knees. The crystals are needle-shaped and so tend to irritate and erode the cartilage, causing inflammation, swelling and acute pain. The first attack often involves only one joint, which is the big toe in more than half of cases. The pain can be extremely severe. In fact a sufferer can often not stand wearing shoes during the daytime, and at night can't even bear the weight of bedclothes on the affected foot.

The first attack may occur at night and is usually preceded by one of the factors that raise uric acid levels. This could be stress, certain drugs (including diuretics) or trauma. However, as uric acid is a by-product of certain foods called purines, gout is closely related to diet. The typical person with gout will be obese, prone to high blood pressure and diabetes, and at a greater risk of cardiovascular disease.

People with gout are typically obese, prone to hypertension and diabetes and at a greater risk of cardiovascular disease

Gout action plan

- Avoid foods rich in purines, i.e. meat, offal, shellfish, herring, sardines, mackerel, anchovies and scallops.

- Avoid fried foods, roasted nuts and fast food high in saturated fats.

- Avoid rich foods such as cakes and pies.

- Avoid refined carbohydrates such as white bread and sugar.

- Eat 6 to 8 helpings of vegetables and fruit (not citrus) daily, to reduce the body's acidity.

- Limit caffeine from coffee, tea, chocolate and diet drinks.

- Eat cherries or drink a glass of cherry juice a day.

- Limit intake of alcohol to prevent the increase in the production of uric acid.

- Drink plenty of water to increase the excretion of uric acid.

- If you are overweight, lose the extra pounds – to lower uric acid levels. But avoid crash diets (and certainly starvation diets) as these may precipitate a gout attack.

- Reduce stress.

- Take up light aerobic exercise or swimming. Exercise helps to increase the circulation and so helps eliminate toxins quicker. Don't forget to drink extra water to replenish lost fluids.

- Discuss any drugs you're taking (e.g. for high blood pressure) with your doctor, in case they've set off your attacks.

Supplements for gout

- Good multivitamin and mineral supplement, particularly if stressed
- Flaxseed oil to reduce inflammation
- Alfalfa, chlorella or spirulina to reduce acidity
- Vitamin C to excrete uric acid

In the acute phase you will need painkillers prescribed by your doctor, and in the longer term you may need drugs to help manage your uric acid levels. Following these recommendations may help you get off these drugs.

Underst
food

Now that you have a better understanding of what your body needs and what can affect it adversely, you can tailor your eating habits to address your specific problems, and bring yourself back to good health. But before doing this, you need to have the basics in place – what makes a balanced diet and which foods provide the nourishment you need so that your body can perform to the best of its ability every day.

anding

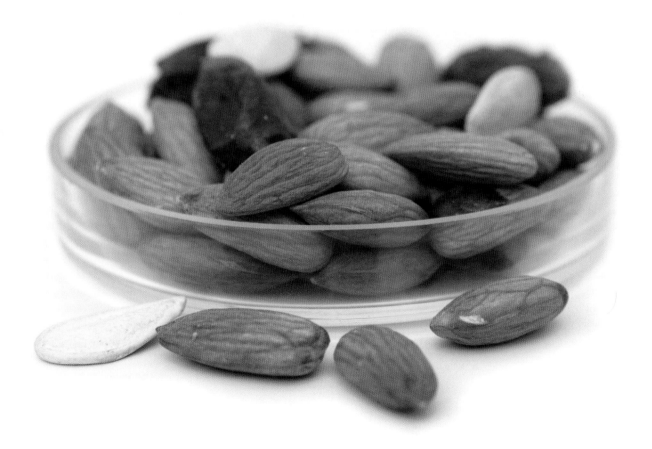

Balancing your diet

How many times have you followed a diet, without fully understanding the difference between a protein and a complex carbohydrate, what each of them do in the body, or in which foods they are found? No dietary plan is ever going to be successful if you don't have the basics in place, so we thought we would lay it out in plain English for you to grasp, once and for all.

In this section we go far beyond the old adage 'an apple a day keeps the doctor away' – we provide the low-down on which nutrients are found in which food, and why your body needs them. In doing so, we provide an invaluable list of the 'angel foods' that are packed with beneficial properties and are essential to a lifelong, healthy diet. We also show how potentially damaging the packet snacks and fizzy drinks can be, and how many of us consume these 'devil foods' without questioning what they contain.

Once you have started eating more healthily, your body will respond rapidly and for the better, and you'll realise it simply isn't worth going back to old habits.

Knowing the food types

All foods are split up into three main categories: proteins, carbohydrates and fats. Some foods can fall into two of these categories – lentils, for example, are a complex carbohydrate, but they also have protein content, making them a well-balanced food for people who aren't eating meat or dairy produce.

Proteins

The word 'protein' comes from the Greek word 'protos' meaning 'first things'. Three-quarters of all the solid matter in your body is protein, which form the building blocks and repairing material for our bodies. Without sufficient proteins, the body actually breaks down faster than it repairs itself.

All animal proteins are complete proteins, that is, they contain all the eight amino acids that the body needs (see next page for definition of the eight essential amino acids). The breakdown products of proteins, amino acids can't be made in the body and must be derived from the food we eat. For vegetarians, most of the proteins contained in grains and pulses are incomplete proteins in that they contain some, but not all, amino acids, and therefore have to be eaten in combination to make up our whole requirement (see Vegetarianism, page 178).

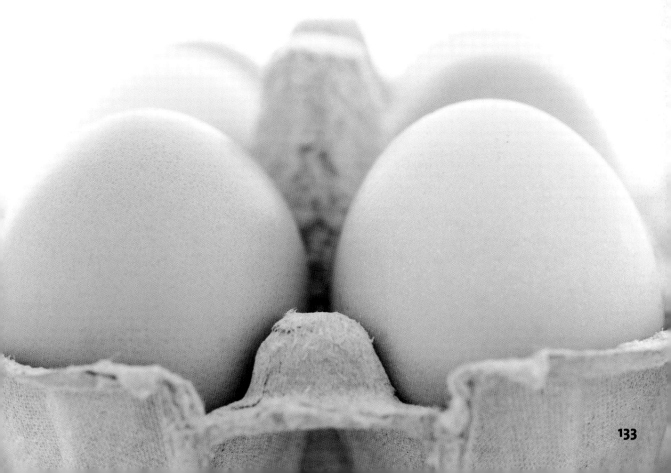

The eight essential amino acids

	Function	Richest sources
Phenylalanine	Used to build insulin and help regulate blood sugar levels. Contributes to the fibrous structures of skin, including collagen and elastin.	Beef, chicken, fish, soya, eggs, cottage cheese and milk.
Tryptophan	Maintains mental function and clarity, relieving depression through increased serotonin production and aids sleep.	Beef, eggs, nuts turkey, cottage cheese and bananas.
Leucine, isoleucine and valine	Used in muscles for building and repair, and aiding wound healing.	Nuts and seeds.
Lysine	Essential for the absorption of calcium from foods. Useful in treating herpes and other persistent viruses. Needed for good skin. Works with methionine to produce another amino acid, carnitine. This helps carry fatty acids into the cells to be burnt, creating the release of energy – a vital function in weight management.	All meats, dairy produce, oily fish and shellfish, eggs, mung beans, chickpeas and hazelnuts.
Methionine	Known as the allergy fighter, also essential for regulating metabolism and energy production (see lysine above). Also required for serotonin, the relaxing mood neurotransmitter.	Primarily meat and dairy products. Also found in sunflower seeds and avocados.
Threonine	Best known for its immune-boosting role, it also helps to deal with inflammatory conditions, e.g. arthritis, eczema and irritable bowel disease.	Wheatgerm, oats, ricotta and cottage cheese.

Proteins should form around 25-30 per cent of the food on your plate (depending on your body type), whether derived from animal or vegetable sources, with adults consuming, on average, just under one gram of protein per kilo of body weight per day. So a 70 kilogram person should consume something in the region of 65–70 grams of protein daily.

While a lack of proteins in the diet depresses all our functions, a long-term high-protein diet places a strain on the body as it causes a high level of acidity. This can be harmful to body tissues. The body, in turn, has several buffering systems to prevent excess catabolism (breaking down of tissue), and will use calcium as a main buffering mineral. This calcium has to be taken out of bones and teeth. Consequently, one of the side effects of a long-term high-protein diet is a higher risk of osteoporosis. This illustrates how important it is to maintain a balanced diet.

Carbohydrates

There are two main types of carbohydrate: complex and simple. Basically, complex carbohydrates are those in wholegrain form, and simple carbohydrates are those that have been processed and broken down before being put back together again. Examples of complex carbohydrates are brown rice, wholegrain bread, porridge oats and muesli, while simple carbohydrates include commercial cereals, white bread, bagels, croissants and biscuits. Most of the simple carbohydrates also have added sugars and often include preservatives, because they are more likely to become stale than their complex counterparts.

The role of carbohydrates is to produce energy. All carbohydrates are broken down into glucose molecules and are the body's preferred source of fuel. In biochemical terms, they go through several stages of being broken down into the simplest of molecules and, with the help of a number of different nutrients (both vitamins and minerals), create energy in the form of ATP (adenosinetriphosphate). This production of ATP is fundamental to a healthy high-performing body, and a deficiency of any of the essential nutrients that go into making ATP will inhibit your body's maximum performance. In order to maintain the body's optimum ATP production, it is vital to choose mainly complex carbohydrates because these are far richer in nutrients and don't have the additives and preservatives that their simple counterparts do.

Balancing blood sugar

Balancing your blood sugar levels is key to maintaining a healthy diet. The body chooses carbohydrates, simple or complex, as its first source of fuel for energy which are all broken down into glucose in the digestive tract and transported in the bloodstream to wherever it is needed at that moment. The more broken down and refined the carbohydrate, (think white flour, white bread, white rice), the faster it releases its sugars into the bloodstream. The pancreas releases insulin to 'carry' the glucose into the organs for energy production, and to keep the blood sugar levels constant.

A quick rise in blood sugar challenges the pancreas to release a high dose of insulin to regulate these fluctuating levels. However, if you live on a high refined-carb diet (commercial cereals and toast for breakfast, sandwich for lunch, and pasta for supper – very common in the West), the pancreas cannot keep up with the demand for insulin, and it starts to respond inappropriately – you experience this as the highs and lows of energy throughout the day, which become progressively more pronounced. This is known as insulin resistance and is the first stage of potentially developing type-2 diabetes. At this stage, adjustments in your diet can help to re-regulate insulin production until it returns to normal. However, if such changes are not made, the fatigue becomes overwhelming and eventually develops into non-insulin dependent diabetes.

Fats

The body needs a certain amount of fats for various vital functions. Remember that the brain is made of around 60 per cent fats, as is the nervous system. All hormones are created out of essential fats and the skin is lubricated and protected by essential fats. Your skin, the largest organ in your body, is your first line of defence so a lack of fats in your diet will actually show first in dry scaly skin, making you look older and more weathered than you are. Let your skin be the tell-tale sign of whether or not you are eating the right kind of fats.

You need to *eat* fat to *lose* fat – mixed nuts and seeds provide essential omega-3 fatty acids which help you to burn stored fat

Saturated fats are found in all meats and dairy produce and are particularly high in cakes, biscuits and patisserie-type treats because they have a very high percentage of butter or vegetable fats. They should be eaten in moderation as they tend to block the action of the beneficial fats, or essential fatty acids, which are required for brain cells and the nervous system.

Polyunsaturated and mono-unsaturated fats are found in nut and seed oils, and are beneficial to the brain and nervous system as well as the heart and cardiovascular systems because they do not block up the arteries. Beneficial fats include olive oil, pumpkin seed oil, walnut oil, nuts and seeds and tahini (sesame seed spread). But to prevent them from turning rancid, they should be kept cool, and not heated. The only oil that should ever be heated for cooking is olive oil. Vegetable oils, which people commonly use for cooking, change their structure when heated, especially when fried at high temperatures, making them potentially damaging to the arteries and cardiovascular system as a whole.

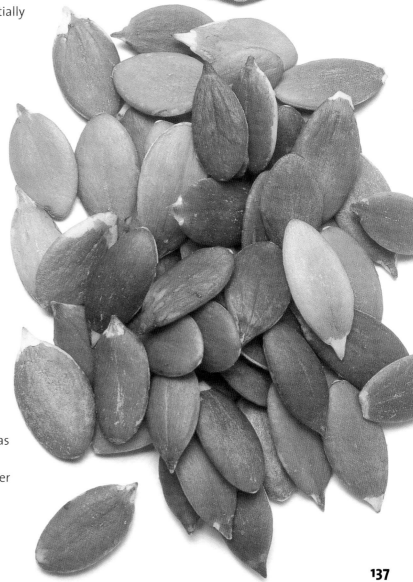

Choose nut oils for added flavour (and essential omega-3 and omega-6 fatty acids) such as pumpkin seed, walnut and hazelnut oils. Use sparingly, as they all have a very strong flavour, and should be mixed with extra virgin or light olive oil.

The omega-3 essential fatty acids that are written about so frequently these days are the best of the essential fatty acids. They are vital for cognitive function and the nervous system, and are responsible for some of the anti-inflammatory processes in the body. They are found primarily in oily fish (salmon, tuna, sardines, herring, anchovies and whitebait), as well as in most nuts and seeds. The best of these are almonds, sunflower and pumpkin seeds.

Vitamins and minerals

Remember, the more varied your diet, the more nutrients you will benefit from, and the better your body will function. There's a world of difference between feeling OK and feeling fabulous, and it all begins here. While we know that vitamin C is good for the immune system, there's so many more vital nutrients that all perform very specific and varied roles in the workings of the body. Listed below are the most important ones to consume on a regular basis.

Vitamins

Most vitamins are water-soluble, that is, they can be absorbed with drinks, fruit and vegetables. However, four key vitamins – A, D, E and K – are fat-soluble and they need to be consumed with foods that contain fats, either essential (as in oily fish, nuts and seeds or their oils), or saturated (dairy, meat, fish, poultry and eggs). Either way, providing you have some protein (either animal or vegetable based, see page 171), with every meal and mini-meal, you will always be absorbing both fat- and water-soluble vitamins.

	Required for	Found in	Deficiency symptoms
Vitamin A (and beta carotene)	Immune system (primary antioxidant), growth and repair of bones, skin, teeth and eye health.	Herrings and mackerel, calves' or chicken livers, egg yolks, dairy produce (vitamin A – retinol), and all red and orange fruit and vegetables (beta-carotene) such as pumpkin, tomatoes, apricots, peaches, mangoes and papaya (paw-paws).	Dry skin, dry and dull hair, hard skin, reduced saliva production, ridged nails that peel across the nail, low sense of smell, loss of appetite, bumps on backs of arms and other parts of the body, acne, mouth ulcers, sinus problems, poor vision at night and poor wound healing.
Vitamin D	Absorption of calcium into bones for strong bones and healthy teeth. Regulates body temperature and works with vitamins A and C to support healthy immune system.	Bony fish (sardines, mackerel, herring, whitebait), and dairy produce and egg yolks. Otherwise synthesised in the body via sunlight through the retina	Misaligned teeth, soft bones, bone and muscle aches and pains, as well as muscle weakness.

	Required for	Found in	Deficiency symptoms
Vitamin E (tocopherol)	Healthy, supple skin, immune system (antioxidant), heart and cardiovascular health, (prevents atherosclerosis, see page 44); helps reduce scarring and improves healing of all tissues.	All nuts and seeds, vegetable oils, eggs, soya beans, oily fish and wholegrains such as oats, rye, brown rice and millet.	Poor wound healing, dry and flaking skin, eczema, palpitations, shortness of breath, anaemia, fatigue, early signs of aging.
Vitamin K	Bone-building and repair, blood-clotting, and preventing heavy menstrual bleeding.	Live bio yogurt and other dairy produce, egg yolks, fish oils and green leafy vegetables.	Easy bruising, osteoporosis and heavy menstrual bleeding.

The B-complex vitamins

The B vitamins all have separate functions in the body, but work best when all are provided. This is especially important when taking supplements – it is recommended that no single B vitamin should be taken without the support of a B-complex multivitamin. Increasing the overall intake of all the foods listed below will lessen the likelihood of any deficiencies.

	Required for	Found in	Deficiency symptoms
Vitamin B1 (thiamine)	Carbohydrate digestion and energy production, heart and cardiovascular function, the nervous system and mental clarity and memory.	Wholegrains including rye, millet, buckwheat, oats and quinoa, as well as legumes, liver and pork.	Depression, poor memory and concentration, lethargy and fatigue, headaches, sensitivity to noise and pain, indigestion or constipation.
Vitamin B2 (riboflavin)	Digestion and metabolism of carbohydrates, fats and proteins, the production of energy, healthy skin, nails and hair, and stress management.	Dairy produce, especially live bio yogurt and cottage cheese, also fish, calves' or chicken livers and green leafy vegetables such as kale, cabbage, watercress and spinach.	Digestive complaints, diarrhoea, constipation, dizziness, insomnia, mental apathy and poor concentration, chapped lips, watery eyes, and scaling around nose, ears and mouth.

	Required for	Found in	Deficiency symptoms
Vitamin B3 (niacin/ niacinimide)	Production of sex hormones (male and female), thyroid hormones regulating metabolism, digestive hormones (including regulation of insulin production and blood sugar management), mood regulation and general nervous system function.	Wholegrains including brown rice, millet, oats and buckwheat. Also green leafy vegetables, egg yolks and dairy produce.	Lowered sexual function and fertility, irritability, fatigue, lack of motivation and concentration, insomnia, dizziness and blood sugar imbalances.
Vitamin B5 (pantothenic acid)	Adrenal glands, digestion and metabolism of carbohydrates and fats, the nervous and immune systems, and healthy ear, nose and throat function.	Wholegrains including wheat, rye, barley and millet. Also nuts, egg yolks, chicken, liver and green leafy vegetables.	Low blood pressure, insomnia, depression, adrenal fatigue, teeth grinding, respiratory infections and constipation.
Vitamin B6 (pyridoxine)	Mood regulation, concentration and motivation, nervous system, growth, healing and repair (works with zinc for these functions). Vital for digestion and metabolism of proteins into energy.	Dairy produce, wheatgerm, chicken, eggs, meat, liver, oily fish and green leafy vegetables.	Depression, PMS symptoms, iron-resistant anaemia, skin conditions (e.g. eczema and psoriasis) and dry hair (including dandruff, scaling of scalp and dermatitis), asthma, diabetes and arteriosclerosis.
Vitamin B12 (cobalamine)	Production of red blood cells (in which iron is carried), cardiovascular health, growth, repair and healing, and good nervous function, particularly focus and concentration.	Red meat and calves' and chicken livers, fish and shellfish, eggs, dairy produce and spirulina (blue-green algae) for vegetarians.	Anaemia, fatigue, restlessness, poor concentration, mood swings, depression and confusion.

	Required for	Found in	Deficiency symptoms
Folic acid (part of the B complex vitamins)	The building of antibodies in the immune system, protein and carbohydrate digestion and metabolism into energy, preventing anaemia, lowering homocysteine levels in susceptible individuals.	Egg yolks, apricots, carrots, pumpkins, squashes, avocados, wholewheat and rye grains and all green leafy vegetables.	Atherosclerosis and arteriosclerosis , anaemia, cracked or sore tongue, poor memory or concentration, fatigue and depression.
Biotin (part of the B-complex vitamins)	Healthy skin, hair and nails, digestion and metabolism of fats and proteins into energy.	Brown rice, nuts, brewer's yeast, calves' and chicken liver, egg yolks and fruit.	Abnormal hair loss, skin complaints (eczema, psoriasis, scaling skin, dandruff), muscle cramps and chronic fatigue.
Vitamin C	Immunity, heart and cardiovascular health, development of sex hormones, stress management, health and repair of skin, both external and internal, and effective wound healing.	All citrus fruits, kiwis, cantaloupes and watermelons, all red berries, squash and pumpkin, sweet peppers, cabbage, broccoli, cauliflower and spinach.	Frequent infections, poor wound healing, skin complaints, fatigue and listlessness, depression, easy bruising, bleeding gums and varicose veins.

Minerals

Minerals are vital to our overall health, working synergistically and tending to stay in the body longer than vitamins. Once any deficiency is rectified, it's unlikely that your mineral levels should go out of balance again, provided you maintain a diet of good fresh food.

	Required for	Found in	Deficiency symptoms
Calcium	Bone-building (in conjunction with vitamins D and C, and iron), heart and cardiovascular health, muscle contraction, good nervous system and healthy ligaments, teeth and nails.	Almonds and other nuts, soya products, green leafy vegetables, dairy produce and bony fish including salmon, sardines, herrings and whitebait.	Muscle cramps, aching bones and muscles, teeth problems and alignment, and soft bones.

	Required for	Found in	Deficiency symptoms
Chromium	The production and support of insulin, regulating blood sugar levels and cholesterol levels in the liver, helping to protect the heart and cardio-vascular system.	Egg yolks, calves and chicken livers, kidneys, wholegrains (all), nuts and seeds.	Sugar cravings, irritability, mood swings, increased PMS, dizziness and energy slumps.
Iron	Formation of red blood cells, carrying oxygen to the brain and other vital organs, growth and development throughout the body.	Calves' and chicken liver, beef, lamb and other red meats, raisins, prunes, dates, figs, apricots, egg yolks, watercress, spinach, parsley, kale and broccoli.	Anaemia, fatigue, muscle weakness, diarrhoea, brittle nails with vertical ridges, dizziness, depression, learning problems and increased infections.
Potassium	Hydration and regulation of fluid content in body, as well as regulating the body's metabolism.	Almonds, hazelnuts, peanuts, lentils and sesame seeds, as well as all green leafy vegetables, particularly watercress, spring greens, spinach, asparagus, kiwi fruits, figs and bananas.	Frequent thirst, pins and needles in the extremeties, cellulite, constipation, palpita-tions, and low or high blood pressure.
Magnesium	Cardiovascular health, nervous system function, stress management, carbo-hydrate digestion and metabolism into energy, thyroid function and mental clarity and function. Also aids absorption of calcium into bones, helps relieve muscle cramps and aids sleep and relaxation.	All green leafy vegetables, citrus fruits, sweetcorn, almonds, other nuts and seeds, mushrooms, figs and raisins, carrots, tomatoes, onions and garlic.	Muscle cramps and twitches, nervous fidgeting, restless legs, hyperactivity and restlessness, insomnia, poor concentration, irritability, palpitations, and arrhythmias. Symptoms are more prevalent in women.

	Required for	Found in	Deficiency symptoms
Manganese	Control of blood sugar levels and energy production, bone health and repair, skin and internal tissue integrity, the nervous system, female hormone production and protection of cells from free radical damage.	Brown rice, lentils, rye bread, oats, buckwheat, quinoa, pecans, walnuts, hazelnuts and macadamia nuts.	Dizziness and irritability. Energy slumps and general fatigue, joint pains, and lowered fertility in women.
Iodine	The production of thyroxine in the thyroid gland to regulate metabolism in the body.	Seaweeds, blue green algae, kelp, seafood (shellfish of all types), and garlic.	Weight gain and inability to lose weight, lowered energy and apathy, constipation, cold hands and feet (even in hot weather).
Selenium	The immune system and most of its functions, the synthesis of natural killer cells to fight cancer, protection of the heart and cardiovascular system, and supporting liver detoxification.	Sesame seeds, peanuts, onions, green and brown lentils, kidney beans, black-eyed peas, chickpeas, shellfish, oysters, clams, crabs, lobster, crayfish, mussels, tuna, trout, swordfish, sardines, mackerel, plaice, cod, calves' or chicken livers and kidneys, sunflower and pumpkin seeds.	Poor wound healing, susceptibility to frequent bacterial and viral infections, chronic fatigue and signs of premature aging.
Zinc	Over two hundred enzyme processes in the body, including many of those involved with the immune system, proper protein digestion, the production of insulin and regulation of blood sugar management, the health and tone of the skin, wound healing, and sperm formation.	Shellfish, mussels, crab, lobster, prawns, crayfish, sardines, liver and kidneys, chicken and turkey, lean lamb, cashew nuts, pumpkin seeds, oats, brown rice, chickpeas, quorn, tofu, quinoa and buckwheat.	Stretch marks and poor or slow wound healing, frequent viral and bacterial infections, colds and flu, aggravated PMS, lowered fertility in men and women, and white spots or flecks on the fingernails.

understanding food

Calories don't count

Calories are the bane of every dieters life. They are the nightmares that haunt every shopping trip and every meal, every day. Yet they have become totally misunderstood and, what's more, misused in the marketing of diet foods in particular.

However, the good news is: counting calories is over! It is an outdated way of calculating what should and should not be eaten, and is often misleading in terms of what is now considered to be a well-balanced diet. Originally designed as a calculation of how much energy a specific food could yield, high calorie foods are now mistakenly used as a warning indicator of how much fat there may be in any specific food. Consequently, many regular dieters are avoiding important foods such as nuts, seeds, oily fish and lean meat, because they assume these foods will make them fatter. But the reverse is true: they will actually improve the rate at which the stored fat in your body can be burnt off, and will ensure you have plenty of energy and concentration.

Manufacturers have cottoned on to the fact that many of us are suffering energy slumps throughout the day, and have conjured up a whole range of foods that are supposedly low-calorie and, at the same time, high energy. Yet it rarely happens that a low-calorie food can provide you with sustained energy. A good example of this is low-calorie commercial breakfast cereals, which consist of simple carbohydrates that release their glucose rapidly – this makes you feel as though you have had an instant pick-me-up. However, these grains have been refined, removing the very grain and fibre that provide all the energy-rich nutrients you need. To combat this, the manufacturer has conveniently replaced those vitamins and minerals in 'added' form to try and put something back, whilst keeping the calories down.

Simply eating a multi-wholegrain muesli or porridge oats will be higher in calories because of their genuine energy-giving nutrients. This is so simple to understand, and yet many are fooled by glitzy advertising claims, promising 'low-fat, low-cal'. What they exclude from the strap-line is that they are also 'low-energy'.

Rather than reading the calories on every label, look at the principles for the PCFF (protein, carbohydrate, fat and fibre) plan according to your Body Type (see page 164) and the Eating for Life food programme (see page 166), and learn how to balance your blood sugar levels to ensure a continuous level of high energy throughout the day. No calorie counting required!

Calories are the bane of every dieter's life, yet they have become totally misunderstood

The Glycaemic Index

The Glycaemic Index (GI) rates the speed at which food is broken down in the digestive tract and its sugars absorbed into the bloodstream and carried to the brain, muscles and other organs for the production of energy. It is simply the amount of energy that is released from that food. It does not relate to calories or fats, but rather to the sugars (simple and complex) that are contained within that food.

All foods and drinks are scored from 1 to 100, with those foods that release their glucose (sugars) most slowly scoring the lowest points, and those that are released quickly, the highest. The lower the GI, the better. Some foods have a different GI according to whether they are raw or cooked. As fibre tends to slow down the release of sugars into the digestive tract, raw food will always have a lower GI than its cooked equivalent, which is one of the reasons why raw food is beneficial for balancing blood sugar levels. For example, carrots, if eaten raw, score a moderate 35 on the Glycaemic Index, but rise to 85 if cooked. Some diets will mistakenly omit carrots altogether because it is assumed that they will always be eaten cooked, and that the GI is too high. Raw carrots (and those that are steamed or only partially cooked) are an excellent source of beta-carotene which is important for the immune system and should not be excluded from any healthy eating plan.

As the Glycaemic Index is used to measure the release of sugars from complex carbohydrates, a specific value is not usually attached to any of the animal proteins. Owing to their protein and fat structure, they all take much longer to digest and release their energy than carbohydrates, and consequently all fall in the low glycaemic index group. Animal proteins (with no specific GI rating) include meats, poultry, fish, shellfish, eggs and dairy produce.

Low GI foods (GI 1-39)

Food	GI	Food	GI	Food	GI
Aubergines	10	Grapefruit	20	Haricot beans	30
Bell peppers (all colours)	10	Soya beans (cooked)	20	Lentils (brown)	30
Broccoli	10	Almonds	22	Milk (semi-skimmed)	30
Cabbage	10	Cherries	22	Peach	30
Garlic	10	Hazelnuts	22	Carrots (raw)	35
Green vegetables	10	Lentils (green)	22	Corn on the cob	35
Lettuce	10	Plums	22	Figs (fresh)	35
Mushrooms	10	Split peas (cooked)	22	Orange (whole)	35
Onions	10	Apples	30	Pears	35
Tomatoes	10	Chick peas (cooked)	30	Plain yoghurt	
Walnuts	15	French beans	30	(semi or full-fat)	35
Apricots (fresh)	20	Fruit preserve (sugar free)	30		

Medium GI foods (GI 40-59)

Food	GI	Food	GI	Food	GI
Fresh apple juice	40	Wild rice	40	Kiwi fruit	50
Fresh orange juice with pith	40	Bulghur wheat	45	Sweet potato	50
		Wholewheat spaghetti	45	Wholemeal bread flour	50
Kidney beans	40	Basmati rice	50	Couscous	55
Peas (green, fresh)	40	Buckwheat flour	50	Shortbread biscuits	55
Pumpernickel bread	40	Brown rice	50	White Pasta (cooked)	55
Rye bread	40	Grapes	50		

High GI foods (GI 60-100)

Food	GI	Food	GI	Food	GI
Banana	65	Sweetcorn (tinned)	70	Carrots (cooked)	85
Jams (sugared)	65	Turnip (cooked)	70	Corn flakes	85
Melon	65	Pumpkin	75	Rice cakes	85
Orange juice (carton)	65	Watermelon	75	Honey	90
Raisins	65	Broad beans (cooked)	80	Potatoes (mashed)	90
Rice (long grain, white)	65	Cheese crackers	80	Chips	95
Chocolate	70	Potato crisps	80	Puffed rice cereal	95
Potatoes (boiled)	70	Baguette bread	85	Rice (pre-cooked, white)	90
Soft drinks	70			Beer	100

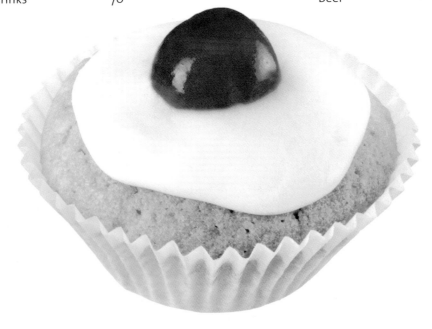

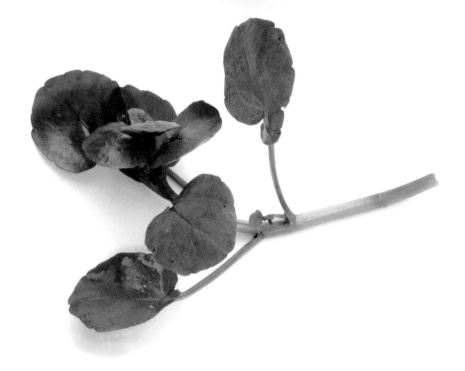

A balanced meal

A more effective way of working out a well-balanced meal is to look at the total combined Glycaemic Index of all the foods on your plate, and work out the average. This is called the total glycaemic load. This does not involve adding up the different weights of foods and dividing or subtracting one from another – it simply means ensuring that if you have a food that has a high GI on one part of your plate (e.g. mashed potato – 90), then you balance that with another food with a low GI (e.g. chickpeas – 30). It's really just another way of ensuring that you combine some protein with some complex carbohydrate at every meal, and reduce or eliminate completely the simple carbohydrates that always have the highest ratings.

For example:
Salmon steak (GI 18) + brown rice (50) + peas (40) + french beans (30) = 138. Divide 138 by 4 = **34.5**. This total glycaemic load represents a well-balanced meal.

On the other hand:
Baked beans (86) + 1 slice white toast (92) = 178 + grilled tomatoes (42) = **220**. Divide 220 by 3 = **76**. This meal is far too high in total and would not deliver long-releasing glucose for energy. Replacing the white toast with wholemeal (45), and eating the tomatoes raw (10), with a slice of ham (20), would bring the total glycaemic load down substantially to (75 divided by 3 =) **25**.

Another prime example of a high total glycaemic load is an Indian takeaway: chicken korma (70) + white rice (50) + onion bhaji (65) = 185. Divided by 3 =**62**. As well as being high in sugar, this whole meal is also very high in fats, and would be better cooked at home, replacing the korma with chicken tikka (no sauce, or added sugar), adding onions to the tikka and baking it all in the oven, rather than having a deep fried onion bhaji.

ANGEL FOODS

All foods that come from natural sources have beneficial properties, but some are considered to be 'angel foods' owing to their exceptional hoard of specific nutrients. The following list of such angel foods shows those that are essential to a lifelong healthy diet – but they should be, by no means, the only foods you eat. The wider the variety of foods eaten on a daily basis, the greater the range of nutrients that you are supplying to your body. What is most important is that you don't eat the same foods day in and day out. Aim to try a new vegetable or fruit every week, and vary your wholegrain intake so that wheat is not the only grain you eat.

Remember that no natural food is 'bad' for you, but some may be considerably richer in their energy-giving nutrients, while others are a good source of antioxidants, and yet others essential for repair and growth.

Fruits and Vegetables

	Source of	Benefits
Apples	Calcium, magnesium, vitamin C and beta-carotene.	Can help to relieve constipation; contain pectin which helps to reduce cholesterol as well as removing toxins from the gut.
Apricots	Calcium, magnesium, copper, iron, vitamin C and beta-carotene.	Natural laxative; iron, calcium and magnesium help to improve circulation; good antioxidant properties.
Artichokes (globe)	Calcium, magnesium, potassium, vitamins B3, C and K and folic acid.	Liver supportive; cholesterol lowering; natural diuretic; blood cleansing.
Asparagus	Vitamins C and K, beta-carotene, potassium, folic acid and asparagine.	Antibacterial; liver supportive and beneficial for kidney health (from asparagine, an alkaline amino acid).
Bananas	Vitamins B6, C, K, beta-carotene, potassium and tryptophan.	Tryptophan helps mood and encourages sleep; B6 is important for mood and mental health; natural anti-fungal, antibiotic; can help to lower cholesterol; also contain pectin which helps remove toxins from the digestive tract.
Beetroot	Calcium, magnesium, potassium, iron, manganese, vitamin C, folic acid.	Excellent liver and gall-bladder cleanser; prevents anaemia; cleanses and stimulates the gut.

	Source of	Benefits
All **berries** (raspberries, blueberries, strawberries, cranberries)	Vitamins C and B3, magnesium, phosphorus, beta-carotene, folic acid and potassium.	Rich in antioxidants which protect against cancer; antiviral and anti-bacterial; raspberries help to dispel mucus; blueberries are a blood cleanser and help to improve circulation; all berries help to support eye-health.
Broccoli	Calcium, magnesium, vitamins C, B3 and B5 and folic acid.	Potent antioxidants, recognised as a prime cancer-preventative vegetable; antibacterial; promotes good peristalsis in the gut; good source of fibre to prevent constipation.
Carrots	Calcium, magnesium, potassium, phosphorus, vitamin C, and beta-carotene.	Good detoxifier of whole digestive tract, liver and kidneys; contain potent antioxidants; naturally antibacterial and anti-viral.
Celery	Beta-carotene, folic acid, B3, coumarin and phyto-oestrogens.	Can help to lower blood pressure, relieve migraines and arthritis; digestive stimulant; female hormone regulator; coumarin contains anti-cancer properties.
Cherries	Vitamin C, calcium and phosphorus.	Relieve gout; anti-spasmodic; natural antiseptic; can help headaches.
Fennel	Calcium, magnesium, phosphorus, vitamin C and potassium.	Good for heart health; aids weight loss as it helps to digest fat and remove excess; natural anti-spasmodic – helps relieve stomach cramp and pain.
Garlic	Calcium, magnesium, sulphur, potassium and vitamin C.	Potent antioxidant; liver supportive (sulphur); reduces cholesterol; heart and circulation tonifier.
Kiwis	Vitamin C, magnesium and potassium.	Help to remove high sodium in the body; good source of inherent digestive enzymes.
Olives	Oleic acid, iron, beta-carotene and vitamin E.	Support liver and gall-bladder health; reduce cholesterol; oleic acid is a potent antioxidant.
Onions	Calcium, magnesium, phosphorus, potassium, beta-carotene, folic acid and sulphur.	Excellent natural antibiotic, antifungal, antiviral, antioxidant; can help prevent and repair stomach ulcers; relieve stomach cramp; liver supportive; detoxifier.
Pears	Calcium, magnesium, potassium, beta-carotene, folic acid and iodine.	Contain pectin which helps remove toxins from the gut; good tonic for cardiovascular health; iodine is required by the thyroid gland to regulate metabolism; natural diuretic properties.

	Source of	Benefits
Peppers (sweet)	Vitamin C, beta-carotene, B-complex vitamins, folic acid and potassium.	Excellent for regulating blood pressure; improve circulation; stimulate production of stomach acid and peristalsis.
Spinach	Iron, beta-carotene, folic acid, B6, calcium and magnesium.	Immune-boosting; blood-building; natural antioxidant; helps to regulate blood pressure.
Squash	Calcium, magnesium, phosphorus, potassium, vitamin C and beta-carotene.	Contains good antioxidants; liver and blood supportive; an alkaline food that settles stomach cramps and acidity.
Sweet potatoes	Calcium, magnesium, folic acid, vitamins E and C and beta-carotene.	Strong antioxidant properties; relieve digestive inflammation; stimulate poor circulation; help to remove toxins from the digestive tract.
Tomatoes	Vitamin C, beta-carotene, lycopene, folic acid, calcium and magnesium.	Lycopene is a potent antioxidant, vital for prostate health; potent antioxidant properties.
Watercress	Calcium, magnesium, iron, beta-carotene, vitamin C, potassium and iodine.	Good for heart, circulation and preventing anaemia; natural diuretic, helps to break down kidney stones; iodine supports the thyroid.

Grains

	Source of	Benefits
Barley	Potassium, magnesium, calcium, manganese, zinc and B complex vitamins.	Energy food; bone-building; lowers cholesterol; relaxes digestive tract; excellent source of fibre.
Brown rice	Calcium, magnesium, iron, potassium, zinc, manganese and B complex vitamins.	High energy-producing food; calming to nervous system; mood regulating; stops diarrhoea.
Buckwheat	Calcium, magnesium, phosphorus, zinc, potassium, folic acid and ruin.	Ruin strengthens capillary walls, important for heart and cardiovascular system; excellent protein source for vegetarians.
Corn	Magnesium, potassium, zinc, iron and vitamin B3.	Relaxing; calming; mood-regulating; good for nervous system and immune system.
Millet	Magnesium, potassium, phosphorus, vitamin B3 and zinc.	Alkaline; calming to nervous system; good source of gluten-free fibre.

	Source of	Benefits
Oats	Calcium, magnesium, iron, phosphorus, manganese, vitamin B5, folic acid and silicon.	High-energy food; excellent bone and ligament builder; prevent anaemia, reduce cholesterol.
Quinoa	Calcium, iron, magnesium, potassium and vitamin B3.	Excellent source of protein; bone-building; supports circulation.
Rye	Calcium, magnesium, potassium, zinc and vitamin E.	Excellent cardiovascular support; alkaline grain that supports the liver and stimulates the digestive system; good source of fibre.
Wholewheat	Calcium, iron, magnesium, manganese, B complex vitamins, zinc and potassium.	High-energy grain; bone-building; supports circulation.

Pulses and Legumes

Chickpeas	Calcium, magnesium, potassium, zinc and folic acid.	High-energy; good source of vegetarian protein; alkaline food that supports kidney health and cleanses the digestive tract.
Kidney beans	Calcium, magnesium, potassium and folic acid.	Good source of vegetarian protein; lowers cholesterol; cleanses the digestive tract.
Lentils	Calcium, magnesium, potassium, zinc, manganese and folic acid.	One of the best sources of vegetarian protein; reduces the lactic acid in muscles after exercise; highly alkaline; regulates digestive function.
Soya beans	Calcium, iron, vitamins C, B3, beta-carotene and omega-3 essential fats.	Contain all eight amino acids making it one of the few perfect vegetarian protein sources (others are spirulina and blue-green algae); regulate female hormones; support heart and cardiovascular health; excellent energy food.

Nuts and Seeds

Almonds	Calcium, magnesium, potassium, zinc, folic acid, B vitamins and vitamin E and omega-3 & 6 essential fats.	Source of vegetarian protein; alkaline; reduce acid stomach; antioxidant protection; good for cardiovascular health and arterial cleansing.
Cashews	Calcium, magnesium, iron, zinc, folic acid, vitamin E and omega-3 & 6 essential fats.	Excellent source of minerals for bone health; good skin-health food; excellent source of vegetarian protein.
Flax/ linseeds	Calcium, magnesium, potassium, iron, vitamins B3 and E, omega-3, 6 and 9 essential fats and phyto-oestrogens.	Stimulate peristalsis in colon; strengthen gut lining; improve bowel movements; regulate female hormones; prevent anaemia; important for cardiovascular health.

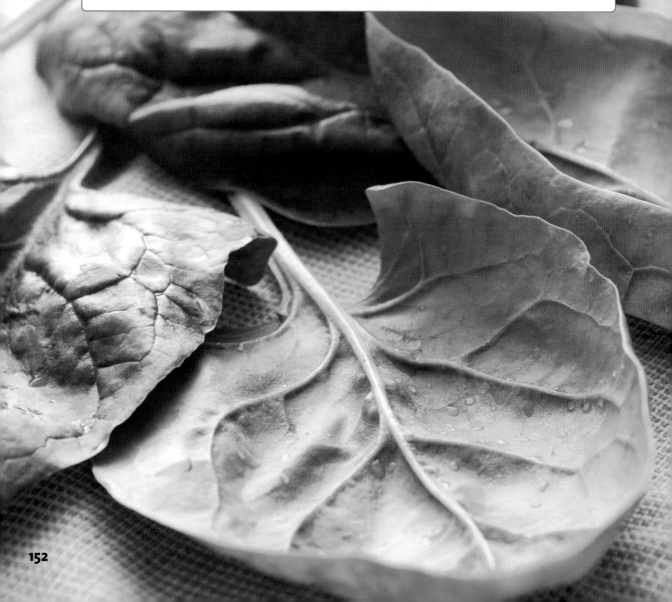

Safe additives

Some E numbers (see page 156) are derived from natural foods and are not only safe, but potentially beneficial. It's worth learning the following list, so that you're not put off a food product that lists only one or two of them, and none of the other potentially harmful additives.

E101	Riboflavin	Found naturally in green vegetables
E160	Carotene	Found in carrots, pumpkin, sweet potatoes, peppers
E300/E304	Vitamin C	Found in citrus fruits, kiwis, tomatoes, broccoli
E306/ E309	Tocopherols Vitamin E	Found in avocados, wheatgerm, seeds, nuts
E375	Nicotinic acid Vitamin B3	Found in brewer's yeast, liver, kidneys, lean meat
E440	Pectin	Found in apples and pears

	Source of	Benefits
Pumpkin seeds	Calcium, magnesium, iron, zinc, potassium, B-complex vitamins and omega-3, 6 & 9 essential fats.	Excellent for prostate health; bone-building; improve skin complaints.
Sunflower seeds	Calcium, iron, zinc, manganese, omega-3 and 6 essential fats, B-complex vitamins, beta-carotene, vitamins A, D, E and K.	A perfect vegetarian source of protein, providing a good source of energy; contain pectin which removes toxic metals from the body; good for improving skin conditions.
Walnuts	Calcium, magnesium, zinc, potassium, folic acid, vitamins C and E and omega-3 and 6 essential fats.	Good source of alkaline protein; potent antioxidant; support kidney health; stimulate metabolism.

Animal proteins

Beef (lean)	Iron, calcium, zinc and potassium.	Important source of iron for regulating anaemia, particularly during menstruation; good source of animal protein in moderation; builds bones, ligaments, hair and nails; repairs organs and tissues; supports immune system.
Chicken	Magnesium, potassium, vitamins A, K, B3 and B6.	Improves mood; provides energy; helps reduce mucus in lungs and digestive tract, soothing digestive complaints.
Eggs	Calcium, iron, manganese, zinc and B-complex vitamins.	Perfect protein, high-energy food; supports bones and joints.
Mackerel	Omega-3 essential fats, selenium, vitamin E and calcium.	Important for cardiovascular health: maintains condition of arteries; cleanses blood; good for improving skin conditions such as eczema and psoriasis.
Sardines	Omega-3 essential fats, vitamin E, calcium and selenium.	Important food for heart health; improve skin conditions; boost immune system.
Tuna	Selenium, omega-3 essential fats, vitamins B12 and B3.	Improves skin conditions; regulates hormones; maintains cardiovascular health.
Turkey	Magnesium, potassium, vitamins A, B3 and B6 and tryptophan.	Tryptophan helps regulate mood and sleep; provides a lean source of energy.
Yogurt (live, bio)	Calcium, vitamin D and acidophilus bacteria.	Supports digestive health; regulates gut bacteria and soothes gut inflammation.

DEVIL FOODS

There are now more fake and synthetic foods available to us than fresh natural foods, and many of the products that start out fresh are tainted with additives, sweeteners and preservatives. This is due partly to the enormous number of foods that the manufacturers churn out every year to entice us to buy more, and partly to our own demands for pre-packed meals and food with a longer shelf-life.

It's important to understand that anything that is added to natural foods will in some way alter their chemical structure, and behave differently in the body. The common habit of running out for a sandwich at lunchtime rarely provokes questions such as, 'How old is this?' or 'How is it that the bread isn't soggy?' We simply take for granted that the ingredients are fresh, therefore the sandwich is okay.

Wrong. In order to ensure longer freshness, the sandwich probably contains a much higher quantity of salt than one that is freshly made in a cafe, and possibly sugar or sweeteners to improve the flavour. It is these ingredients, and many more synthetic versions, that are causing so much of our current ill-health and obesity. Such ingredients are designed not only to enhance flavour but also to create cravings for more of the same.

Addicted to junk

It's nothing new in our culture to be addicted – one way or another – to nicotine, alcohol or recreational drugs. What is new, and growing at an alarming rate, is an addiction to fizzy drinks and junk food, as well as a reliance on processed food that may not be wholly 'junk' but is infinitely inferior to the fresh variety.

As people eat more and more 'synthetic' and 'altered' foods, the inherent nutrients of such foods are either insufficient or out of balance. Couple this with the fact that a lot of popular foods are almost completely devoid of any nutritional value, and it's no wonder that so many people develop cravings. A good example is a typical commercial breakfast cereal. Already completely stripped of its fibre, it will lose most of the minerals and almost all of the vitamin values as it's processed to crisp or flake, to the point that nutrients have to be added back into the product to justify any health claims at all. However, while this kind of food is a poor way of delivering nutrients, it's not necessarily addictive.

On the other hand, the soft drinks and snacks that form a daily part of many people's diets contain an abundance of sweeteners, emulsifiers, colourings and other chemicals that may be addictive in the long term – replacing vitally important foods, and robbing the body of important nutrients.

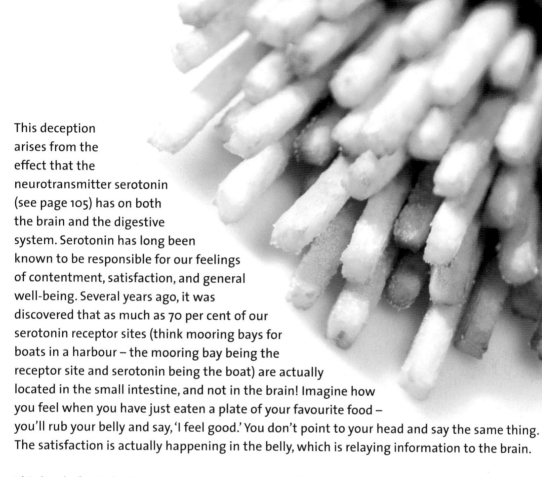

This deception arises from the effect that the neurotransmitter serotonin (see page 105) has on both the brain and the digestive system. Serotonin has long been known to be responsible for our feelings of contentment, satisfaction, and general well-being. Several years ago, it was discovered that as much as 70 per cent of our serotonin receptor sites (think mooring bays for boats in a harbour – the mooring bay being the receptor site and serotonin being the boat) are actually located in the small intestine, and not in the brain! Imagine how you feel when you have just eaten a plate of your favourite food – you'll rub your belly and say, 'I feel good.' You don't point to your head and say the same thing. The satisfaction is actually happening in the belly, which is relaying information to the brain.

This level of satisfaction tends to occur more quickly with synthetic foods and drinks, because the chemicals in these reach the brain and have the effect of distorting the balance of serotonin/dopamine, and you are conned into thinking it 'makes you feel good'. Unfortunately, this feel-good factor doesn't last very long because it is unnaturally produced, and you are left feeling low and needing another 'fix'.

In addition, most of these types of foods contain sugars, or sugar replacements, and other unnatural stimulating chemicals that actually produce a stress reaction in the body. The adrenal glands release adrenalin (see page 92), which we experience as a rush of energy, or increased heat in the body, or both. This stimulating effect can make us feel good – energized and ready to go – a sensation that can easily become addictive.

Sadly, these 'enhanced' foods are insidious in their addictive nature. That is, you probably don't even realise how addictive they are until you try to stop eating or drinking the offending food. The most common example of these are the diet fizzy drinks, which contain nothing natural other than water – see page 159.

Demon E numbers

Listed below are the common E numbers that form part of our daily diets. Note that many of these are found not just in quick-snack foods and fizzy drinks, but also in many of the pre-packed ready meals that form a large part of the western diet. The inclusion of an E number indicates to the consumer that these ingredients are considered safe for use, but do not warn of any side effects in specific conditions, other than ADD or hyperactivity in children – and there has been very little research into the potential harm from combinations of E numbers.

Sweeteners

Many of these are used in products that claim to be sugar-free. They are frequently found in diet drinks, chewing gum and no-sugar confectionery. The side effects are often mild, but cumulatively could be far more damaging. In many cases, the long-term effects are largely unknown. Some of these are many times sweeter than the sugars they replace, but tend to become as addictive, with added hidden side effects.

Number	Name	Linked to
E951	Aspartame	May cause dizziness, blurred vision, migraines
E954	Saccharin	Bladder cancer
E950	Acesulfame-K	Cancer links
E420	Sorbitol	Diarrhoea, flatulence, laxative
E421	Mannitol	Nausea, vomiting, diarrhoea
E422	Glycerol	Headaches, thirst, nausea, high blood sugar levels

Other sweeteners, which have no designated E numbers, include:

Sucralose	Bladder cancer
Glucose/Fructose syrup	Obesity and type-2 diabetes
Xylitol	Dizziness, nausea

Flavour enhancers

These are frequently used in low-salt products to comply with the government-regulated levels of salt/sodium. Unfortunately, many of them tend to cause more serious side effects than the salt they are replacing.

E622	Potassium hydrogen glutamate	Nausea, vomiting, cramps
E627	Guanosine	Nausea, breathing difficulties
E631	Inosine	Nausea, stomach upset, itching
E621	MSG – monosodium glutamate	Effects range from mild dizziness to unconsciousness; breathlessness and asthmatic reactions

Colours

E102	Tartrazine	Skin rashes, insomnia, breathing problems
E104	Quinoline	Hyperactivity, aggression, asthma
E107	Yellow 'G'	Asthmatic reactions, hyperactivity
E110	Sunset Yellow	Serious stomach upsets, urticaria, hyperactivity
E120	Cochineal Carminic acid	Hyperactivity, aggression
E122	Carmoisine	Hyperactivity, oedema, urticaria
E124	Ponceau	Asthmatic reactions
E129	Allura Red	Skin sensitivity
E131	Patent Blue	Nausea, low blood pressure, tremor, hyperactivity, urticaria – reaction can be immediate
E132	Indigo Carmine	Vomiting, nausea, high blood pressure, skin rashes, itching, breathing problems
E133	Brilliant Blue	Hypertension, hyperactivity
E154	Brown FK	Asthma, skin rashes, urticaria
E155	Brown HT	Asthma, aspirin sensitivity, hyperactivity

Preservatives

The following preservatives are commonly found in many products that have a shelf-life of anything from five days to three years. These additives form the largest group of all and are particularly problematic to those who already suffer breathing or skin conditions. The easiest solution is to exclude them all from your diet, although it is worth noting those that appear to be related to symptoms from which you frequently suffer.

E200	Sorbic acid	Possible skin irritant
E210	Benzoic acid	Asthma, urticaria, gastric irritation, hyperactivity or anxiety
E211	Sodium benzoate	Asthma and urticaria
E212	Potassium benzoate	Allergic reaction for asthmatics
E218	Methyl 4-benzoate	Anxiety, allergic reactions affecting skin and mouth
E219	Methyl 4-hydroxy benzoate	Skin irritations, anxiety, numb mouth
E220	Sulphur dioxide	Asthma, anxiety, hyperactivity
E221	Sodium sulphite	Asthmatic hypersensitivity
E223	Sodium metasulphate	Asthmatic hypersensitivity, anxiety
E224	Potassium pyrosulphite	Asthmatic hypersensitivity, hyperactivity
E226	Calcium bisulphite	Gastric irritation, asthma, skin reactions, hyperactivity
E230	Biphenyl	Nausea, vomiting, ear and nose irritation
E239	Hexamine	Gastric and urinary upsets, skin rashes
E251	Sodium nitrate	Hyperactivity
E252	Potassium nitrate	Abdominal pain, vertigo

The sweetener blues

One of the staggering facts about sweeteners is that, gram for gram, they are actually much sweeter than sugar itself, and the average 500ml fizzy drink contains the equivalent of six to eight teaspoons of sugar. When you also take into account that just one teaspoon of sugar lowers the function of the liver by 50 per cent, for up to six hours, you start to wonder how on earth it survives.

Sugar can have a seriously disruptive effect on the body, and no one questions it because it is found in virtually everything we eat. The major disruption it causes is to the blood sugar levels and the production of insulin. This increases the risk of type-2 diabetes, as well as encouraging more unhealthy snacking and eating. Frequently, those who drink several fizzy drinks daily become low in mood and lacking in motivation, as the chemicals challenge the natural balance of the brain's neurotransmitters, such as serotonin and dopamine (see page 105), which are vital to our general sense of well-being.

One of the most disturbing aspects of the fizzy drink trend is that it is often drunk in combination with alcohol, creating the new craze of alco-pop binge drinkers. The mix of alcohol and very sweetened drinks is a lethal cocktail, with effects very similar to those of recreational drugs. Many young people are left in a state of mind that leads them to behaviour they wouldn't otherwise engage in – young women are especially vulnerable.

People on diets drink a lot of fizzy drinks, particularly those who have eating disorders such as anorexia and bulimia – since the diet varieties list no calories at all. This is hardly surprising, when the only natural ingredient to be found is water. The rest of the ingredients are all chemical, aimed to create a specific taste and fizz. Imagine the effect this might have on someone who is not eating more than a piece of fruit and a lettuce leaf throughout the entire day, and nothing more than a few cups of tea, to keep them going. The main effect is on the brain chemistry, which exacerbates the feelings of anxiety and obsession. It is critical that such drinks are removed from the diets of obsessive eaters, as they simply compound the problem and are ultimately more addictive.

Remember the Golden Rule: Fresh is best

The trouble with fizzy drinks

The fizzy drink industry has grown faster than any other sector of the market over the last 15 years, overtaking all natural options, such as fruit juices and bottled spring waters. With the increase in dieting, the consumption of fizzy drinks in place of meals or snacks is all too common. The long-term effects, however, are rarely considered. The additives in the drinks tend to leach valuable nutrients, particularly minerals, from the body in a similar way to caffeinated drinks. Calcium is used to buffer the potentially harmful effects of such high levels of sweeteners on the liver and kidneys, affecting bone density and the health of teeth and gums.

Fizzy drinks are, effectively, a stressor to the body, causing repeated stimulation of the release of adrenalin and cortisol from the adrenal glands. This may leave you feeling initially uplifted, then subsequently fatigued. The quantity of sweeteners frequently causes headaches, irritability, loss of concentration and focus, as well as desires for foods with a similar taste.

Quick-fix packet snacks

Vicki says: 'I believe these to be the devil of all devils as they have become, for many, the mainstay of the daily diet, replacing fresh fruits and raw vegetables. The combination of crispy texture with salty taste becomes irresistible to those who consume them regularly, and manufacturers compete endlessly to produce the ultimate mini-meal. Yet the preservatives and flavourings used in such snacks are known to cause high blood pressure, anxiety and altered blood sugar levels. They are also notoriously high in hydrogenated fats, to replace saturated fats found in their fresh alternatives such as cheese, meat and seafood. They temporarily suppress the appetite, and are therefore perceived as being good meal replacements for those who are dieting. How much more can consumers be deceived by such a diabolical concept?'

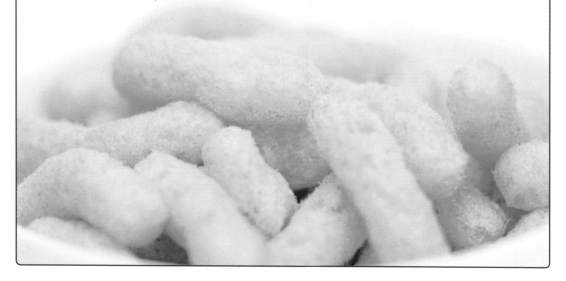

Eating

With a broader knowledge of which foods do what in your body, the burning question now is: how do I put it all together? The answers are actually very simple, and they are all laid out here. We show which foods suit your body type, how to balance and portion your food correctly, and what to avoid if you're on a specialist diet. Your aim should be to develop a new relationship with the food that you put in your body for health and vitality now and for the rest of your life.

for life

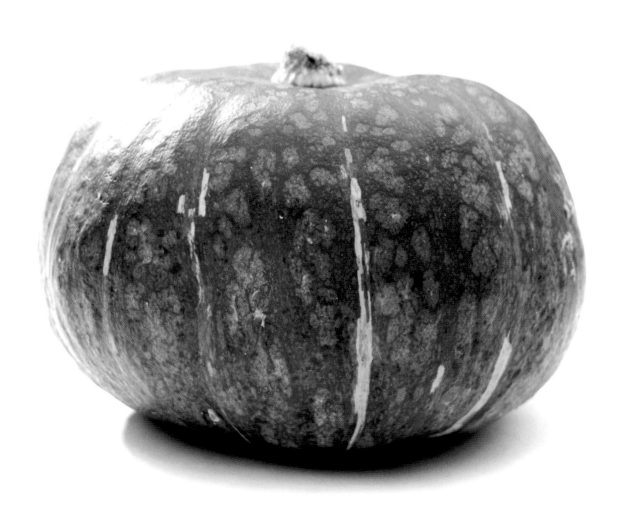

Take control

If you were to keep a food diary for a week, you would probably find that you eat many of the same foods daily, and you rarely choose alternatives simply because it's easier to prepare foods that are familiar to you. But familiarity breeds boredom, and with that comes excess or inappropriate choices.

The average person in this country eats only 30 to 40 different foods in any given week, when they could be eating between 120 and 140. Think of all those vital energy-giving nutrients that you are missing out on with such a limited choice. Never before have you been blessed with such a variety of foods on offer, so give yourself the best chance of balancing all your body's requirements and try to eat as varied a diet as possible. Be adventurous, and see how quickly your body responds. This challenge ensures that you are making many more fresh food choices, rather than resorting to easy-fix prepared meals or fast foods.

The beauty about our Eating for Life food programme is that it is not restrictive, it invites you to enjoy a much more positive attitude to your food and mealtimes, and you can experience the benefits of healthy eating within a matter of weeks. You'll never turn back.

Diet *(noun)*: fare, nourishment, nutrition, sustenance

Interestingly, given the dictionary definition of the word, 'diet' has been misused, taken to mean 'cutting down', 'cutting out', 'limiting' or 'reducing', when in fact the original meaning was about providing the right foods in balance and harmony. The notion has developed that if we eat all the food groups (i.e. proteins, carbohydrates, essential fats), we shall inevitably put on weight, and that only by cutting out or restricting one or more groups can we lose weight. This is simply not true.

The most popular recent diet plans – the Atkins Diet (high protein, high fat, low or no carbs), the F-Plan (high fibre, low fat, low protein), and the Protein Power (high protein, low carb and medium fats) – all advocate a major group that should be favoured and a second group that should be omitted or greatly reduced. Such an approach may seem to work at first: omitting any one food group will inevitably create a rapid initial weight loss as the metabolism has to adjust itself in order to adapt to the foods that are being provided for fuel. As energy is the primary requirement for the body as a whole, it will start to break down its own fat stores, and subsequently its own lean tissue, to provide that energy in the absence of the correct foods in balance.

But such diets can work only in the short term – they simply cannot be sustained as the body requires all three food groups in order to function properly. This is why fad diets don't work; they ultimately create cravings for the very foods that have been restricted or cut out completely, simply to supply the body with all the nutrients it needs. Sadly, many people will swing from one diet to another, hoping to find the one that will suit them. They are permanently either 'on a diet' or eating badly in between. This is known as yo-yo dieting and serves only to upset the metabolism, making it more difficult to lose weight. And as they swap from one dietary approach to another, they inevitably cut progressively more foods out of their diet altogether.

And one kind of diet will by no means fit all. If we all ate the same foods, in the same ratios, would we all be the same size, and put on and lose weight in the same way? We know this isn't the case. The key here is the difference in body types, each of which has different dietary requirements.

Determining your body type

Three main body types have been identified, although there are many subtypes. For the purposes of this book, the focus is on the three main types, although you may feel that you are part of more than one type. Where this is the case, you should follow the dietary recommendations for the type that is dominant. Your body type is determined by the waist-to-hip ratio, or WHR. To determine your WHR:

+ Measure the circumference of your waist and then the circumference of your hips.

+ Divide the first number by the second.

+ If the answer is in the range 0.72–0.78, you are an endomorph.
  If the answer is in the range 0.82–0.89, you are an ectomorph.
  If the answer does not correspond to either of the above ranges, you may be a mesomorph.

Your waist-to-hip ratio should not be greater than 0.9 for men and 0.85 for women. A ratio greater than this can predispose you to heart disease, osteoarthritis and diabetes.

Mesomorph

This is the 'string bean' shape: the shoulders and hips tend to be virtually identical in width with a fairly straight/boyish waist. String beans can eat a broad range of foods without readily putting on weight, and can lose it more easily than Apples and Pears when they do. They have longer legs, and overall are well proportioned. They are often athletic, able to build muscle well, and also respond to lengthening exercises such as yoga and pilates.

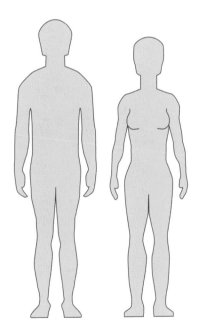

String beans fare best on a well-balanced diet of wholegrains, animal and vegetable proteins, fruits and vegetables. They can also eat larger amounts of nuts and seeds than the other shapes, as they use the essential fatty acids in them without putting on weight. They can eat more shellfish, too, as they are not prone to high cholesterol, and they suffer less risk of cardiovascular disease. Happily, they rarely need to diet, providing they don't eat junk food.

Regardless of body type, the risk of developing life-threatening disease is higher if you are overweight.

Endomorph

This is the 'pear' shape: wide hips and thighs, flatter or droopy bottoms, and narrow shoulders, with weight gain always occurring in the lower body. Pears therefore appear to be bottom-heavy, with short legs. They have a lower risk of heart disease than Apples, even when their BMI (see page 14) is high.

Pears crave high-fat foods and dairy foods in particular (cheese, butter, cream and ice-cream) and have little interest in fresh fruit and vegetables. Yet it is important for Pears to lower their saturated-fat intake and regulate their blood sugar levels (see page 136), and include plenty of vegetables to increase their fibre intake.

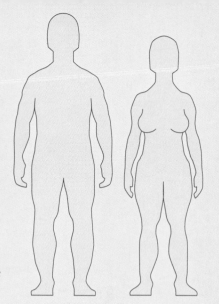

Ectomorph

This is the 'apple' shape: a broader upper body and smaller lower body, with weight gain tending to occur around the middle. Apples are most likely to gain weight, but are also able to lose it with the correct dietary changes and regular exercise. However, the risk for heart and cardiovascular disease, with high cholesterol, is higher in Apples than in the other shapes. Most significantly, 85 per cent of women with diabetes are apple-shaped; they also have the highest risk of metabolic syndrome (see page 98).

Apples tend to crave simple carbohydrates, such as white bread, potatoes, biscuits and cakes. They are usually plagued with a sweet tooth and are most commonly overeaters and bingers. It is important for them to cut out all refined carbohydrates and replace with complex carbs and wholegrains only. Studies have shown that Apples who change their diets to include 20 or more servings of wholegrain foods per week can cut the risk of developing heart disease and stroke, as well as type-2 diabetes, by 40 per cent.

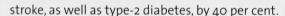

If Apples increase proteins in their diet, with plenty of vegetables (5 to 6 portions a day), they're likely to regulate their blood sugar levels well. However, they should keep their consumption of fresh fruit to no more than 2 to 3 portions a day, as the sugars in these tend to cause sweet cravings.

Soya products are particularly beneficial to Apples, as favouring the intake of soya replaces the saturated fats found in dairy produce, with the added benefits of the phytoestrogens that can help to regulate female hormones. Essential fatty acids found in nuts and seeds also benefit Apples (no more than 30g per day), as they are an excellent source of vegetable protein to replace some of the animal proteins that are high in saturated fats, and make a good snack to help to regulate blood sugar levels in between meals.

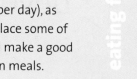

eating for life

While your body type is a useful guide, no diet will work if you don't stick at it. All too often a serial dieter will pursue an eating plan for no more than six or seven weeks before giving up, going through a period of bingeing, and then embarking on a new approach, only to fail again. Rather than a quick-fix, short-term approach, what you need is a healthy, lifelong programme that maintains your diet in the true sense of the word.

The Eating for Life food programme

The mainstay of the Eating for Life food programme is to ascertain what percentages of each of the food groups you should be eating, according to your body type (see pages 164). A simple system allows you to continually check if you are eating the right foods in balance. This is called the PCFF system:

P – Protein

C – Complex carbohydrates

Fa – Essential fats

Fi – Fibre

Fibre is added to the three main food groups because, while most complex carbohydrates include fibre, it is of the soluble type – that is, fibres that create bulk in the intestines, and help to carry out toxins and other residues with the stool. Also important to include are the insoluble fibres that are found in fruits and vegetables – think celery stalks, apple skins and sweetcorn. These fibres are not broken down entirely, and serve to act as the intestines' natural toothbrush, cleaning and sweeping as they pass through. It is vital to consume both types of fibre as each performs different functions in the gut.

Unfortunately, many diet plans opt for omitting the starches (i.e. wholegrains, cereals, breads, potatoes and other root vegetables) as many of them are delivered in a more refined form, which delivers their energy more rapidly (see Glycaemic Index, page 145). This means that those carbohydrates containing so many of the B vitamins, vital for the production of energy, are reduced. Other sources of such fibres and B vitamins are found predominantly in pulses and legumes, but these do not suit everyone's digestion. Therefore these wholegrains and cereals are important to retain.

First, check that you have identified your body type (Apple, Pear or String bean).

Next, look at the chart opposite for the ratios of PCFFs you should be consuming every day.

Then familiarise yourself with the Angel Foods, check out the Golden Guidelines and then turn to the Recipe section (pages 198-219) for guidance on how to achieve this.

Finally, check portion control!

Note: There is no calorie-counting involved in this system – it is simply about getting the balance of the food groups right.

Apples

Apples require a higher ratio of lean proteins than either Pears or String beans, as they tend to store their weight around the middle. They also need a good percentage of both types of fibre to ensure that they don't become constipated.

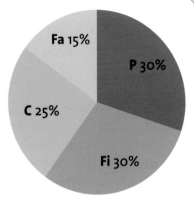

Pears

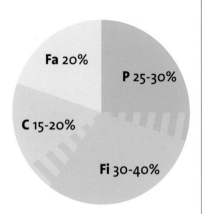

Pears require a higher ratio of complex carbohydrates and are particularly well suited to beans, pulses and legumes. They need to keep their consumption of animal proteins low as they tend to store their fat in the hip and thigh areas which they find difficult to shift, so it is vital that they consume plenty of fibre.

String beans

String beans have the most flexibility with their percentages, as they don't put on weight as easily as Apples and Pears, and have a more even weight and fat distribution. They can consume the highest ratio of lean animal proteins of all the groups, and function best eating plenty of fibre and relatively low complex carbohydrates.

There is nothing radical about this system – there are no major omissions, other than to cut out all junk food, and to ensure that 80 per cent of the food you eat is fresh and in its natural state. This allows for 20 per cent of your daily consumption to include foods you may already tend to eat, which may be delivered in a more convenient form, for example a ready-prepared supermarket soup (still fresh, but not homemade). This ratio is the first of the golden guidelines (see page 170). It allows you the flexibility to eat out, to eat at friends' houses, and to eat abroad without feeling like you have 'come off the programme'. This is the secret to its success: no guilt, no failure, just guidelines.

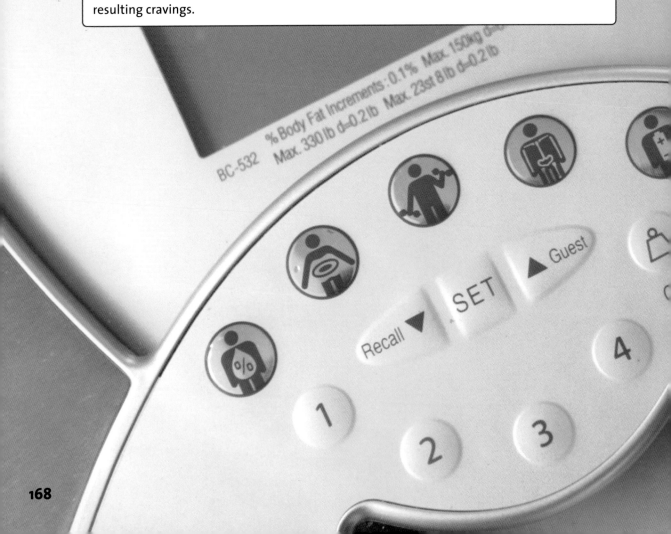

How much, how quickly?

Much research has gone into this subject and there seems to be a consensus that long-term steady weight loss is safer, and likely to be more permanent, than any quick-loss diet. Across the board, it has been found that an average of 2lb or 0.8kg per week is the optimum weight loss that will encourage changes in metabolic rate that, crucially, can be sustained. Most quick-loss diets will promise up to 10lb in the first week, which is more often than not merely loss of fluids rather than fat.

This means that, over the course of six months, it is possible to lose upwards of 3 stone, or around 21kg. And, most importantly, this loss can be permanent. (For the more seriously overweight or obese it is possible to lose more than this in the first 3 to 4 months, as much of the weight initially lost is due to inflammation of tissues and stored fluids.) There are no fad diets that can promise the same thing without causing major nutrient deficiencies and resulting cravings.

Kicking the junk habit

If you've been in the habit of consuming foods high in synthetic additives, then you may well have developed something of an addiction to them (see page 154), which will make it more difficult to keep to the Eating for Life food programme. Don't try to cut out the offending foods all at once – it will be more effective to wean yourself off them gradually. Having said that, you should avoid all fizzy drinks, and other high-sugared products right from the start. In fact, don't touch any diet product that contains sweeteners, as these are, effectively, mood-altering. The worst of these is aspartame, a sweetener used in many foods and drinks, and particularly those that are bright orange coloured (see E numbers, page 156). These can be the greatest offenders, and progress is rarely made in the long term until these types of food and drink have been removed from the diet altogether.

On the positive side, the obvious first step is to eat the kind of wholefoods listed in this section. They contain a range of nutrients that genuinely feed your mind and body and once you start, the cravings for synthetic food will lessen almost immediately. A good start would be replacing all simple carbohydrates with complex varieties such as brown rice, wholegrain breads and muesli/porridge rather than refined cereals.

In addition, it is vital to balance your blood sugar levels (see page 136), so that you're supplying yourself with the correct balance of foods to alleviate cravings when you're tired.

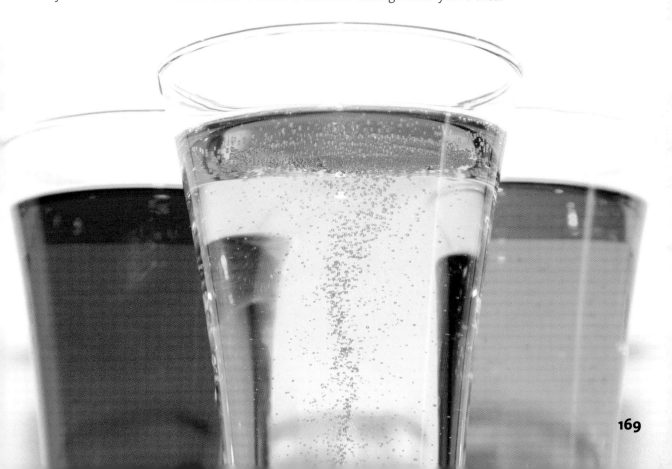

The golden guidelines

These main principles are to be followed 80 per cent of the time. This is known as the 80/20 rule.

+ You don't need to follow any diet or restrict the number of daily meals, even when you just want to lose a few extra pounds – you simply eat less for a week or so, but you keep the balance of food groups the same and follow the Eating for Life food programme.

+ You always follow the PCFF – protein/complex carbohydrate/good fats/fibre – distribution on your plate at every main meal, rather than counting calories.

+ You eat little and often, ideally not less than every 3–4 hours, whether a main meal or a snack to keep your blood sugar levels balanced. Never go all day without a meal. You'll simply eat too much at the end of the day.

+ You don't wait until you are starving to eat – you will only make inappropriate choices.

+ You aim to choose fresh and wholefoods for at least 80 per cent of your meal planning, trying new and seasonal foods to increase the variety and keep you interested.

+ You will choose to avoid all 'fake' and 'fast' foods and fizzy drinks at any cost – knowing that these devil foods will simply lead you down the slippery path to old habits and weight gain.

+ You aim to develop a new relationship with the food you put in your body, increasing your knowledge of what you need and what you don't.

+ You eat only those foods you enjoy, not forcing yourself to eat anything just because you know it to be healthy. It may well be healthy, but it may not suit you.

+ You will give yourself credit for the hard work and commitment that you put into this plan. You will not give up when and if you slip off the slope, but simply pick up where you left off.

Eating for life

Just to show you how wide the variety of foods available to you are on the Eating for Life food programme, we have created below a comprehensive list of the recommended proteins, (animal and vegetable), carbohydrates and foods containing all the beneficial fats to inspire you. Next, turn to the recipe section. Be adventurous – it's so much more stimulating to the taste buds to try new foods!

Animal protein

Poultry	Fish	Shellfish	Lean meats	Dairy products
chicken	tuna	shrimp	lean beef fillet	milk and hard cheese (goat, ewe and cow's, for variety)
turkey	herring	scallops	young lamb steaks and cutlets	feta and halloumi
game birds (e.g. pheasant, grouse, duck, partridge, quail)	mackerel	lobster tails	ham off the bone	crème fraîche (instead of cream)
eggs from chickens and game birds	sardines	crayfish	veal	plain organic bio yogurt
	salmon	clams	calves' liver and chicken liver	frozen yogurt with fresh fruits
	halibut	mussels		
	cod	crab		
	sea bass			
	sea bream			
	red mullet			
	grey mullet			

Vegetable protein

Pulses and legumes	Soya products	Nuts	Seeds
lentils	fresh soya beans (edamame), steamed	almonds	sesame
split peas	soya milk and plain soya yogurts, with fresh fruits	hazelnuts	sunflower
kidney beans		walnuts	pumpkin
chickpeas		pecans	flaxseeds (linseeds)
garbanzo beans	tofu	cashews	poppy seeds
butter beans	tempeh, barley or brown rice miso	pine nuts	seed butters and oils
haricot beans		nut butters and oils	
aduki beans			
pinto beans			
black-eyed beans			
broad beans (fava beans)			
black beans			
pigeon peas			

One of the most effective principles for weight loss, and subsequent management, is to restrict the consumption of starches (grains and relevant vegetables) to daytime meals only. An excess of them in the evening will not be used for energy, and may be converted into stored fat. Choose a maximum of two portions of grain-based starch and one vegetable-based starch each day, to ensure that you maintain the correct PCFF balance through the day.

Grains (starches)

Wholegrains	buckwheat	millet	red rice	bulgur wheat
barley	quinoa	wholewheat	wild rice	triticale (a mix of wheat and rye)
oats	corn (maize)	sprouted wheat and wheatgerm	brown basmati rice	popcorn (popped)
rye	polenta (rough-ground maize)	brown rice	couscous	
spelt				

In cereals, breads and crackers	oatbran flakes	millet pancakes	wholewheat pitta bread	corn crackers
porridge	rye bread	buckwheat pancakes	gram flour flatbreads (naan, Lebanese flatbreads)	brown rice crackers
granola	wheatgerm bread	corn (maize) tortillas		rye crispbreads
muesli	wholewheat muffins	cornbread	oat cakes	
wheatbran flakes	oatbran muffins			

In pastas and noodles	corn pasta	buckwheat noodles (Japanese soba noodles)	brown rice noodles
buckwheat pasta	durum wholewheat pasta		

Starchy vegetables

These are mainly root vegetables, and they tend to have a higher glycaemic index (see page 145) when cooked – that is, they release their sugars relatively quickly. Some starchy vegetables may be eaten raw, but on the whole they should be cooked and combined with extra protein to slow down the release of glucose into the bloodstream to balance blood sugar levels. Do not eat these with your evening meal, to prevent conversion of starches to stored fat.

acorn squash	corn (on the cob)	parsnips	leeks
butternut squash	potatoes	carrots	green peas
pumpkin	sweet potatoes	Jerusalem artichokes (not globe)	okra
beetroot	turnips		

Non-starchy vegetables and herbs

These may be eaten throughout the day as well as in the evening meal since they don't upset the blood sugar levels in the same way as the starches.

asparagus	cabbage	endive	mustard greens (mustard and cress)	sugar snaps
artichoke (globe)	carrots (raw)	fennel		snow peas
beansprouts	cassava	garlic	onions	shallots
beetroot tops (greens)	cauliflower	ginger root	parsley	spinach
bell peppers (all colours)	celeriac	green beans	pumpkin flowers	spaghetti squash
borage	celery	kale	courgettes	Swiss chard
broad beans	chicory	kohlrabi	mange tout	tomatoes
broccoli	chives	lettuce	radishes	turnip greens
Brussels sprouts	cucumber	mushrooms	radicchio	string beans
	eggplant (aubergine)		rocket	watercress

Fruits

The two basic rules when choosing fruits are: indigenous and in season. It is best to eat mainly those fruits that are grown in the same continent in which you were born, to reduce the likelihood of intolerances and digestive upsets. Regard foreign fruits as a treat and they will benefit you – be greedy and you're guaranteed an upset digestive system!

apples	red or white currants	kiwi fruit	tangerines	pomelo
apricots	dates	kumquats	papaya (or pawpaw)	quince
avocados	elderberries	lemons	passion fruit	raisins
bananas	figs	limes	peaches	raspberries
blackberries	gooseberries	lychees	pears	rhubarb
blueberries	grapefruit	loganberries	pineapple	strawberries
boysenberries	grapes	mangoes	plums	tamarind
cherries	Cape gooseberries	melon	pomegranates	tomatoes (green yellow and red)
crab-apples	guavas	mulberries	prickly pears	tomatillos
cranberries	jackfruit	nectarine	prunes	watermelon
		oranges		

Fibre

Very simply, your fibre is found in all the grain-based carbohydrates and in all fruits, vegetables and salad foods. In order to ensure an adequate amount of fibre on a daily basis, you should include at least one grain-based portion and four to five based on vegetables and fruit per day. Eating more portions of vegetables is encouraged, but don't eat more than 3 portions of fruit per day, as this will throw your blood sugar levels out of balance.

How big is a portion?

Vicki says: 'There are a number of different guidelines suggesting the 'correct' size of a portion of food, including those recently issued by the Food Standards Agency. In my opinion, none of these takes individual size and weight into account, and I fail to see how a 26-stone man can be recommended to eat the same amount as a 14-stone woman, even if both are trying to lose weight. I therefore prefer using a combination of two methods: the palm method and the one-plate method.'

The palm method

The size of our hands is relative to our height and ideal weight. It makes sense therefore to use them as a means of measuring the size of portion relevant to yourself.

Cup your hands together, as though they're the bowl you'll serve your food in, and look at the total area they create. You can use this total size for servings of the carbohydrate portion of any main meal:

+ A salad (without the protein content)
+ A total serving of all the vegetables you might eat with your main course
+ A bowl of cereal, muesli or porridge
+ A plate or bowl of pasta (buckwheat, corn or wholewheat)
+ A plate of risotto (brown rice – see recipe page 208)

Now look at the size of your palms – you can use them to measure the portion size for protein at any main meal:

+ Poached or scrambled eggs or an omelette – 2 or 3 eggs depending on your size
+ Fish steaks (halibut, cod, hake, salmon and tuna) – one palm
+ Fish fillets (sea bass, dover sole, lemon sole, plaice) – both palms across
+ A slice of cheese (not a chunk!) – one palm
+ A portion of tofu, lentil dhal or Quorn slices (for vegetarians) – one palm

Eating fast foods and those that are 'super-sized' gives us permission to eat far more than we actually need.
Ask yourself – 'Do I *need* this, or am I simply eating because it's on my plate?'

The one-plate method

Very few people pay attention these days to the size of the plates and bowls they serve their food in, although there used to be very specific sizes of plates for different courses of food, which afforded a more realistic measurement of how much should be sitting on them. In fact, it has more recently become fashionable to serve food in oversized plates to make the food look attractive, arranged in the middle, but as time has elapsed this has simply allowed more food to be served in larger plates, and consequently the correct portion has become distorted.

A side plate is usually 6 or 7 inches (15–18cm) in diameter, without its rim, and a dinner plate is 9 or 10 inches (20–22cm). Therefore, a starter should be served on a side plate and a main course on a dinner plate. It is worth your while to check your plate sizes so you can accurately work out how much you should be having on your plate, and not allowing your hunger or greed to override the serving size.

The most important rule about the one-plate method is to serve yourself just one plate, and accept that is the total size of your meal, no matter how delicious it is. If you want to lose weight, you are going to have to impose certain restrictions on your usual portion sizes, and this is one of the simplest ways of doing just that. So a main meal would all be served on one dinner plate, or partially on a dinner plate, with a side salad or extra portion of vegetables on a side plate.

Equally, the size of your breakfast bowl or bowl for main-meal soup or salad should have a relative measurement. Some people prefer a deep bowl for their morning cereal and others a shallow soup bowl, which usually measures 7 or 8 inches (18–20cm) in diameter, without the rim. Either is suitable, but remember that a single bowl of either type is sufficient for your total breakfast, or as a starter of soup for a main meal.

Oversized plates allow more food to be served, and consequently the correct portion has become distorted

Combining the one-plate and the palm methods

A breakfast, for example, could consist of a bowl (either shape) of porridge, with a dessertspoon of mixed nuts and seeds and a palmful of fresh fruits. This would all fit into one bowl. Having this fulfils all the criteria for PCFF (proteins, carbs, essential fats and fibre), and should be sufficient for most people. However, if your palms are quite small, you may need to adjust how full your bowl is. It is a good idea to look at your favourite meals that you eat most frequently, and actually measure out the amounts you should be having, as though someone else were serving you. Be honest with yourself – have you been more than over-generous of late? You will find that, within a short time, you realise that you are satisfied with the correct serving size for you, providing you are getting your proteins and carbohydrates in correct proportion.

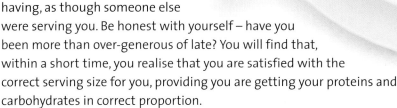

Oils for cooking

Vicki says: 'Whatever the portion size, and however the food is cooked, I recommend no more than 1 dessertspoon of light olive oil per person. So, if you are fry-steaming (as in stir-frying, but adding stock, water or wine to the dish), you need no more olive oil than if you are marinating a piece of fish to be grilled, i.e. one dessertspoon.

'For salad dressings, the temptation is often to use more oil than vinegar or citrus juice, which produces an over-dressed salad. Top chefs maintain that you should never use so much dressing that you can't taste the individual leaves and salad components. As a nutritionist, I would insist that you do not use an excessive amount of oil for health reasons, and would recommend extra virgin oil for dressings.'

Specialist diets

Choosing a specialist diet for some is a luxury, whilst for others is a necessity. If it has been determined that you have a food intolerance (see page 69), you may wish to omit those particular foods from your diet for several months, or even permanently until the related problems have subsided completely. We recommend that you work with a qualified nutritionist or integrated medical health practitioner to make sure you aren't missing out on vital nutrients (such as amino acids in vegan diets, and calcium in dairy-free diets).

Vegetarian

The number of vegetarians has risen sharply in the UK in the last 15 years, and there are now an estimated 3 million people (5 per cent of the population) who are following a mainly vegetarian diet. Some still eat eggs, milk or cheese, but no red meat, chicken or fish. Pescatarians are those vegetarians who eat no kind of meat, but who do eat fish and shellfish; they account for about 2 per cent of the whole population.

While some ethnic groups follow a vegetarian diet as a tenet of their faith, and other people do so as a matter of animal-rights principle, many have 'converted' as a result of food scares concerning meat, most recently BSE and 'human mad cow disease' – also known as Variant Creutzfeldt-Jakob Disease. A vegetable diet is seen as healthier – and there is a valid reason for that: naturally enough, it encourages the consumption of more fruit and vegetables. However, vegetarians should steer clear of ready-packed foods, and make sure they vary what they buy. Most vegetarians consume only about 0.4g of protein per kilo of body weight per day, only half the recommended amount for the average adult. it's therefore important that they grasp the principles of proteins (see page 133) and amino acids, and how they work in the body.

Another risk in the vegetarian diet is anaemia. Most people know that this is caused by a lowered level of haemoglobin that gives red blood cells their colour, and transports oxygen and iron around the body. This is one of the reasons why vegetarians often appear pale in complexion. What isn't so well known is that it can also be the result of low levels of vitamin B12

Vegetarians need a good selection of pulses, beans, and soya-based foods to get all the essential amino acids

Refined wheat 'treats' (biscuits, crackers, doughnuts) cause cravings that often get out of control

and folic acid. Folic acid is found in many fruits and vegetables, as well as some pulses (see angel foods, page 148), but B12 is less available for true vegetarians as it is found mainly in red meat, poultry and saltwater fish and shellfish. For vegetarians it is found only in seaweeds, and blue-green algaes such as chlorella and spirulina. These are best taken in dried powder form, and added to soups and breakfast smoothies (see recipes, page 199).

Vegan

A vegan diet is even more limited than a vegetarian diet as it forbids eating any food that comes from an animal, or any animal by-product (eg. eggs, milk, cheese). Veganism is increasingly popular in adolescents and young people who are concerned about the hormones and antibiotics that are fed to dairy cattle and other sources of meat. However, care must be taken to ensure that adolescents are not using veganism as a method of food restriction. Following a macrobiotic diet (designed for vegans) is complex and limiting, and vegans often lack essential B vitamins that would normally be derived from animal-based products. It is advisable to seek professional advice if such a diet is to be followed in the long-term to prevent potentially harmful deficiencies.

Wheat-free

Over the last few years, wheat has become almost a dirty word. It's true that the western world has developed an addictive tendency towards foods made from refined white flour, which sadly bears few nutrients, rendering them as 'empty calorie foods'. With such a cheap ingredient, manufacturers are able to create an endless array of cereals, pastas, biscuits and other sweet treats at very low cost. These refined-wheat products tend to cause bloating and wind in the gut, as well as creating an almost glue-like paste in the intestines when combined with the mucus secretions and digestive enzymes that normally play such an important function in the process of digestion and absorption.

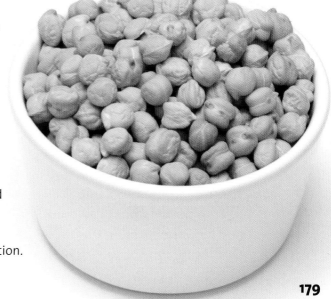

Generally speaking, it's recommended that you cut out all processed wheat foods from the diet when weight loss is a concern to encourage the consumption of more nutrient-rich foods. Wholewheat grain does appear in the angel foods (page 150) as this variety of wholegrain includes many essential minerals, vitamins and fibre – all needed for balancing blood sugar levels, lowering insulin production and creating a well-balanced diet.

For a small number of people, wheat can create inflammation and other intolerant reactions, particularly for those who suffer from irritable bowel syndrome (see page 70) and depressive illness. The best way to assess if you are intolerant to wheat-based products is to cut them out of the diet completely for three to four weeks and see if you feel significantly better.

Alternatives to wheat

Cereals
Oats, millet flakes, barley, buckwheat (not a grain specifically, but part of the rhubarb family), rye flakes and quinoa are all good choices. Porridge or muesli can be made from a combination of any of these alternatives, according to taste.

Pasta and noodles
Dried buckwheat or corn pasta is the best alternative to the usual durum wheat pasta, but rice pasta is somewhat tasteless. Rice noodles (the brown rice variety), on the other hand, are a good addition to vegetable and protein stir-fries. The best choice is soba (buckwheat) noodles that are both rich in nutrients and filling. They form the basis of many Asian dishes, which are easy to adapt at home (see recipe on page 204).

Biscuits and crackers
Rye cakes, oat cakes, corn and rice crackers are all readily available in supermarkets, but it is important to select those that have not been salted, or coated with synthetic flavourings. Oat and fruit bars abound, but some are very high in sugars – best to make them at home.

Flours
Traditionally, wheat flour is used for baking, and for thickening sauces. It is just as effective to use other flours, but many of them are not as strong as wheat, so it is advisable to find a cookbook that specifically deals with this type of baking. Maize, millet, buckwheat, gram (chickpea) and barley flours are all good alternatives, and form the base for many traditional Middle Eastern flatbreads. Rice flour is too fine for breads and muffins, but may be used as a thickening agent.

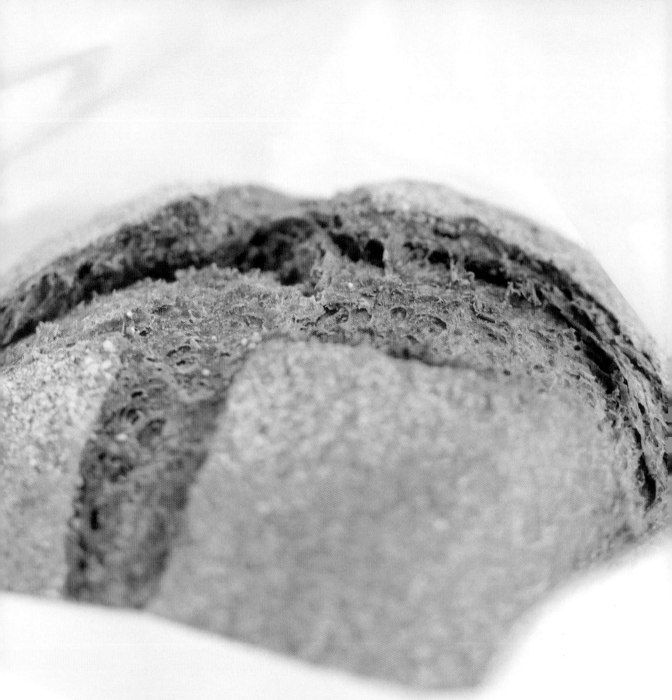

Fifty years ago every woman knew how to bake bread – what happened to that knowledge of basic, wholesome nutrition?

Gluten-free

A small number of people are gluten-intolerant or even gluten-allergic. Coeliac disease is the name given to a severe reaction to all grains that contain gluten (wheat, oats, rye and barley). Gluten (or gliadin) is the protein part of the grain, which can cause severe diarrhoea and extreme weight loss. It is rare to get beyond childhood without this condition being diagnosed, since it is usually present from birth, but it may also be triggered by surgery, trauma, severe food poisoning, or long-term stress.

In all events, it is vital to remove all gluten grains from the diet completely and, in some cases, all grains, but this should be undertaken only after appropriate testing and under medical supervision, or with the help of a nutritionist.

Dairy-free

Dairy produce is a major part of a child's diet in the western world, as it contains important minerals, including calcium for bone-building. However it forms no part of the Asian or Afro-Caribbean diets.

In adulthood, the enzyme that is required to digest dairy produce (lactase) is often reduced or even non-existent, and it is thought that as the human species evolved, we required only mother's milk during our early years and no further dairy produce of any kind in adulthood. This would explain why some people find that while they enjoyed dairy products in childhood, they subsequently cannot digest them in later years.

If you think you may have a lactose intolerance you should undertake a blood test. The two main components of milk are whey and casein, and tests will indicate which creates the intolerance. Either way, it is strongly advisable to opt for a dairy alternative for several weeks to ascertain the degree of sensitivity. Many skin complaints are related to dairy intolerance.

Symptoms of lactose intolerance include abdominal bloating, wind, stomach cramps and diarrhoea

Those who suffer from severe digestive diseases such as Crohn's and ulcerative colitis should definitely remove all dairy products from their diet, as should those people who suffer from irritable bowel syndrome. If you think you may be reacting to cow's dairy products, it is a good idea to remove them from your diet and consume only goat's and ewe's milk and cheese. Goat's milk is closest to human breast milk in its composition, providing almost the same quantities of essential fatty acids, while cow's milk contains much less.

There is now an abundance of dairy alternatives, available in supermarkets and specialist health-food shops. Try some of the following, which are much lower in their allergenic tendency:

+ Rice milk
+ Soya milk
+ Oatly (made from soaked oats)
+ Almond milk
+ Hazelnut milk
+ Combination milks – soya, nuts and grain

The nut milks are especially beneficial to vegetarians, as they contain many of the essential amino-acids; you could make your own nut milk by soaking oats in water overnight, then blending the soaking water with the oats or the nuts until smooth. The less water, the more creamy the consistency.

The joy of soya
Soya milk and related products have become increasingly popular as a dairy alternative, and it is interesting to note that in Asian countries, where no animal dairy produce is eaten, soya is a staple part of the diet. Coincidentally, the countries that include soya in their daily diet have a lower rate of obesity, female hormone-related imbalances and hormonal cancers. This is due in part to the phyto-oestrogens (phyto = plant based) that are found in soya beans, that help to balance any overproduction of oestrogens produced in the body naturally. Pears (endomorphs) are particularly well suited to the change from dairy to soya.

The importance of removing dairy products from your diet is critical if you are suffering from obesity, high cholesterol or any other cardiovascular condition. This is because they constitute the highest saturated fat content after red meats.

The only dairy product that may be considered in a totally dairy-free diet is organic live plain bio yogurt. This contains Lactobacillus acidophilus, the beneficial bacteria found naturally in the gut to fight infections and pathogenic bacteria found in foods that have been reheated or poorly prepared. You should consider including this only after you have completed the three-week total exclusion approach.

Clear out the junk

It's time to take stock of your larder – clear the shelves of all the junk that seemed a good idea at the time and make sure the only food you stockpile is what will contribute to the best, healthiest and tastiest diet of all. So get rid of these:

+ Cakes, biscuits and high-sugar snacks

+ Lo-fat products (that have high sugars)

+ Fizzy drinks, including diet varieties

+ Sugar-free chewing gum

+ Brightly coloured chewy sweets

+ Commercial, sugared cereals

+ Refined breads (white, croissants, baguettes, bagels)

+ Crisps and other packet snacks

Stocking the larder

Although food in its fresh state is the ideal, a well-stocked store cupboard is essential. Don't consider it a cop-out, rather it shows good planning. A carefully chosen mix of dried, tinned and bottled foods , as well as flavourings, gives variety to the diet and makes you more versatile in the kitchen – as well as saving you time. And when you come home tired to an empty fridge, you'll always have a supply of excellent, nutritious food to hand – from fish to pasta, beans to noodles – which will keep you away from fast-food snacking.

You could copy these next two pages and keep them with you as a shopping list, so that you can top up the essentials on a weekly basis. Or you could create your own list of choices, remembering to vary them regularly so you don't fall into the trap of eating the same foods week in and out.

Grains

Jumbo oats, millet flakes, buckwheat flakes (home muesli mix)

Quinoa

Bulgur wheat

Couscous

Pearl barley

Brown rice

Carnaroli risotto rice (Italian, white wholegrain rice)

Red Camargue rice (from France, red in colour, and rich in nutrients)

Wild rice (black wholegrain)

Muesli (unsweetened)

Rye crispbreads

Corn crackers

Wholewheat pasta

Corn pasta

Buckwheat pasta

Rice noodles (dried)

Nuts and seeds

Note: all nuts should be unsalted and raw, not roasted, and stored in the fridge from purchase (not once the packet has been opened) to prevent rancidity, and increase shelf-life.

Almonds

Cashews

Pecans

Walnuts

Sesame seeds

Pumpkin seeds

Sunflower seeds

Poppy seeds

Linseeds (flaxseeds)

Nut butters

Use these in moderation rather than peanut butter which is very high in saturated fat.

Almond nut butter

Cashew nut butter

Hazelnut butter (but not chocolate varieties!)

Pulses and legumes

All pulses, beans and lentils may be dried or ready to use in tins.

Lentils (puy and red)

Chickpeas

Borlotti beans

Kidney beans

Black-eyed beans

Butter beans

Cannelini beans

Flageolet beans

Tins, bottles, jars and cartons

Anchovies in olive oil

Herrings in oil or brine

Salmon in brine

Sardines in olive oil

Tuna in brine

Artichoke hearts

Olives in brine or olive oil

Passata tomatoes (skinned, deseeded and puréed)

Tomatoes, chopped, with herbs

Tomatoes, plain chopped

Olive oil, extra virgin (for dressings)

Olive oil, light (for cooking)

Pumpkin seed oil

Sesame oil

Walnut oil

Cider vinegar

Red wine vinegar

White wine vinegar

Wholegrain mustard

Honey

Low-fat coconut milk

Herbs and spices

Bouquet garni

Oregano

Rosemary

Sage

Thyme

Allspice

Chilli powder

Cinnamon (sticks or ground powder)

Coriander (seeds and ground powder)

Cumin

Garlic paste

Ground ginger

Harissa paste (Moroccan spices)

Nutmeg (whole or ground)

Paprika

Star anise

Turmeric

Vanilla essence

Vanilla pod

Wasabi paste (Japanese)

Lo-salt or potassium salt

Vegetable stock powder (lo-salt varieties only)

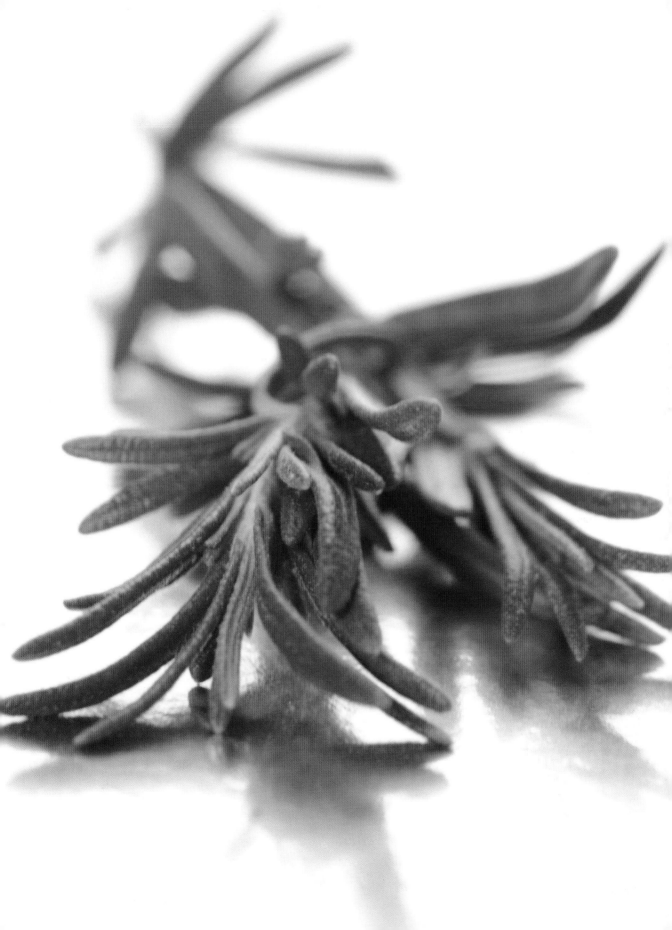

Fit for Life
Get moving

Mention the word exercise and most people want to reach for chocolate cake. There's something about that word and its connotations of gyms, breathless running or crowded aerobics classes that puts many people off even attempting to lose weight.

The good news, however, is that you don't have to make yourself feel sick through exertion in order to lose weight. Simply put, you need to get off your bum and start moving! If you're overweight, then you may already think you're active because you're almost certainly exhausted by the end of the day. Carrying around excess weight is always tiring and puts a lot of extra strain on your body. But be really honest with yourself now – do you walk up stairs or always take the lift? How many car journeys do you take door to door, when really you could walk at least part of the distance? Maybe you even send an email when you could walk across the office to deliver the message in person? If you really sit and think about it, how active are you during the day?

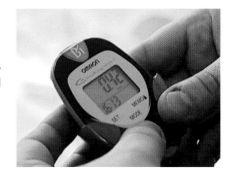

Almost every major function in our bodies depends partly on exercise for its optimum function – our digestion and elimination, our lungs and breathing, our heart and cardiovascular system and not least of all our weight management! Government guidelines recommend that every adult should aim to walk at least 10,000 steps per day. For those without pedometers (and if you haven't got one they are highly recommended) that equates to 90 minutes' walking for the average person. It might sound a lot but 50 years ago this would have been the norm for every one of us. Today most overweight people are often walking less than 3000 steps per day and it's estimated that we now eat between two and three times as much as we did 50 years ago. No wonder we are a larger nation!

You may not have an excessively outrageous diet, but if you're not moving, you will put on weight. It's a simple mathematical equation – calories in versus calories out. You can try all the latest diet crazes around but in the end your success or failure will boil down to how you balance this simple equation.

Get walking

Quite simply, walking is essential to your health. It exercises virtually all your muscle groups, with all the major muscles being used at the same time, providing you aim to walk at a brisk pace and swing your arms to help propel you along.

Walking increases your heart-rate (pulse) and ensures that blood is being pumped round your body at a faster pace than when you are sitting still. The heart itself is a muscle, and needs imposed exercise. Anyone with a cardiovascular condition is encouraged to 'get moving' and to take aerobic exercise at least four times a week. Cardiovascular exercise is any activity that increases the heart rate to its maximum (HRM). Ideally, you need a heart rate monitor for this, which you can purchase from any sports shop. Alternatively you can go by your breathing. When you're out of breath, you are most likely at your HRM (see below). Once the breathing is lower you can increase intensity again.

✚ Heart rate maximum test

A heart rate monitor consists of a band that is wrapped around your chest or ribcage and a device that reads your heart rate. Once you've programmed in your age and gender it will calculate your heart rate maximum (HRM) and flash when you have reached it.
Your **heart rate maximum** is calculated as follows:

> **Women:** 220 minus their age = HRM
> **Men:** 226 minus their age = HRM

For example, a 40-year-old woman would be about 220 minus 40 = 180 (HRM)

Walking also improves your lung capacity (size of lungs, and their full use) and depth of breath. Many of us only use shallow breathing in our everyday lives, that is we are breathing down into the first third of our lungs only. We use the peak flow test to see how well our patients are breathing (see page 57). Walking and other high intensity aerobic exercise (swimming, cycling, skipping, running) all force the need for a deeper breath and better use of the lungs. As well as improving lung capacity, it also ensures better waste clearance from the lungs (oxygen in, carbon dioxide out).

Digestion, particularly elimination, is improved with walking and other aerobic exercises – many people who have very sedentary lifestyles have constant constipation. The body was designed to move and when our overall movement is limited, so too is the peristaltic action in the large intestine (muscular action that moves faecal matter through the bowel for elimination). Walking, in particular, encourages the whole of the digestive tract to move consumed food through the system. Optimum digestion occurs when we are erect (standing), when we are breathing properly (i.e. fully into the lungs), and when the cardiovascular system is working to full capacity. That does not mean that you should go for a brisk walk immediately after a meal – on the contrary, wait at least 40 minutes after eating before enjoying any cardiovascular exercise. This does not apply if you are simply walking to work after breakfast, as you will not be aiming to reach your HRM, but rather you will walk at a steady pace all the way.

A natural high

Walking is also the perfect antidote to depression and anxiety. It can aid the release of serotonin which is why many people experience a natural high and lift in mood after exercising. Walking can also enable people to feel closer to their loved ones because they get a chance to talk to partners, children or friends rather than being distracted by the television or the internet.

Skin benefits

In addition, walking will encourage the elimination of waste matter through sweating, which is an important elimination process that sedentary people rarely experience. Our skin is the largest organ of elimination, and our bodies depend on this method to prevent the internal build-up of toxins. Skin will look cleaner and clearer within a couple of weeks of aerobic exercise, including walking, with more colour in the cheeks and a healthier glow.

How to stretch

Before any form of exercise it's very important to stretch to protect yourself from injury. This is particularly crucial if you haven't exercised for a long time or are overweight.

+ The neck

Hold each stretch for ten seconds. Standing or sitting upright, slowly turn your head to the right until the muscles start contracting in the neck. Then turn to the left and hold again. Turn the head facing forward, look up and extend the neck backwards. Then bring the head forward and tuck the chin into the neck, hold, and release.

+ Shoulders, chest and arms

Standing or sitting upright, place both arms behind the back. Interlock fingers with palms facing each other. Slowly raise your straight arms away from the body. Hold for 10 to 15 seconds, keeping neck upright, and relax.

+ Back of upper arms and upper back

Stand or sit with one arm straight out in front of the chest. Grab the upper arm just above the elbow with the other hand, and pull across the body. Hold for 15 seconds, then repeat with the other arm.

+ Back, upper and lower legs

Standing upright, slowly bend your upper body towards the floor with hands pointing in the direction of the toes. Don't force the movement, but try to get as close as possible to the toes. When muscles are stretched fully, hold for 10 to 20 seconds. Straighten up slowly. To start, stand with your feet shoulder-width apart. As your flexibility improves, move feet closer together for an increased stretch.

+ Front of upper and lower leg

Stand upright and bring one foot towards your buttocks by bending the leg. Grab your ankle with your hand and pull the foot against your buttocks. Keep your balance for 10 to 20 seconds, then repeat with the other foot.

+ Back of thigh

Sit on the floor with your upper body nearly vertical and your legs straight in front of you. Lean forward from the waist and reach towards the toes with your arms. Keep looking forward and toes pointing up. Hold for 20 seconds and then relax.

+ Calves and back of lower leg

Stand with the heel of one foot 8–9 inches (15–20 cm) in front of the toes of the other foot. Bend the front ankle forwards with the heels still touching the floor. Lean forward, and try to touch the front leg with your chest. Hold the stretch for 10 to 20 seconds, then repeat with the other leg.

✚ The three-minute step test

This is a fitness assessment test that measures the heart rate in the recovery period following three minutes of stepping. If you can't finish the test, or score at the Very Poor level, you should check with your doctor that it's safe to continue. Do not attempt this test if you're taking beta blocker medication (or any other medication affecting heart rate).

Equipment

- ✚ 12-inch (30cm) step
- ✚ Stop watch (or watch displaying seconds) for timing test and counting recovery heart rate
- ✚ Metronome to set cadence (may use pre-recorded audio cassette tape and player)

Procedure

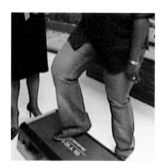

- ✚ You must first stretch (see page 191).
- ✚ Then step up and down at a rate of 24 steps per minute (metronome setting of 96) for three minutes.
- ✚ Immediately after the three minutes, sit down and find the pulse at your neck. Five seconds after you stop stepping, count your heart rate for 60 seconds.

This recovery heart rate is the score. Consult the chart to determine your fitness category.

Fitness category	Gender	Heart Rate
Excellent	male	under 71
	female	under 97
Good	male	71-102
	female	97-127
Fair	male	103-117
	female	128-142
Poor	male	118-147
	female	143-171
Very Poor	male	over 148
	female	over 172

The 4 x 20 fat burner miracle

+ **Do you have little time for exercise in your present lifestyle?**
+ **Do you get bored with your present exercise regime, or hours of cardiovascular exercise?**
+ **Have you never previously had good results from your cardio regime in the past?**

If you answer yes to any of these questions, then the 4 x 20 fat burner is for you. You will never outgrow this simple regime and it will always remain effective. Despite what many trainers advocate, low-intensity, long-duration cardio workouts are not the best method for losing excess fat. Research has shown that *high-intensity* training burns fat more effectively and more efficiently.

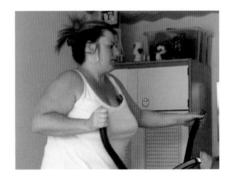

How the programme works

It involves doing 20 minutes of aerobic exercise two to three times per week. Your goal is to make each workout the most effective fat-burning, health-enhancing 20 minutes you can. In every workout, you have to have four peaks of intensity. That means increasing your intensity to the point where your heart rate increases to its maximum.

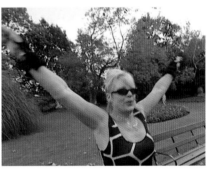

The great point to understand about this programme is that you can do *any* form of exercise that you choose, as long as you can increase your intensity to the point where you reach your HRM (see page 189 to determine your heart rate maximum) – e.g. swimming, cycling, running, skipping or steps. Do note that steps achieved during these workouts should be included in your daily step count.

Hours spent in the gym is not the answer – your body needs a short, sharp challenge for effective weight loss

fat or life

When and how to walk

You can walk at any time and build up to your 10,000 steps cumulatively throughout the day. Here are some suggestions:

✚ At work, walk the last two flights of stairs, rather than taking the lift.

✚ Wake up and go for a 15 minute brisk walk before having your shower in the morning. Yes, it does mean waking up 20 minutes earlier, but it will be worth it – try it and see!

✚ If walking your dog, move faster and stay out for 10 minutes longer than you do at present.

✚ Walk to the shops – don't drive. If it means you have to shop more often, because you can't carry all the bags, so much the better. The more trips done, the more weight you'll burn off, and the more attentive you'll be about WHAT you are filling those bags with!

✚ Walk home from work, or at least the last 20 minutes of your journey. You may feel tired, but it will give you some time to leave your work behind and create some space between work and home life – you will actually arrive home feeling more energised, rather than more tired.

✚ When travelling or shopping, walk up the stairs instead of taking the escalator.

✚ Allocate one of your days off (weekend or otherwise) to enjoy a really good walk – in the park, countryside or somewhere other than where you walk on a daily basis. Time to reflect, plan ahead, and breathe fresh air is almost as good a tonic as a holiday. Try it once and you'll be doing it every week.

✚ Wear loose clothing – nothing creates more uncomfortable sweat than tight clothing. If you are heavily overweight, they will also create friction where skin and clothing rub together, such as on the thighs and upper arms.

✚ Wear good quality trainers. Cheap or inadequate trainers for walking (especially on long walks) can contribute to shin strains, Achilles heel problems and fallen arches. If this is the first investment you make in your health, you won't regret it. Good trainers are vital.

If you have finished reading this section of the book, put the book down, put your trainers on, and go for a good walk – you'll see how just this simplest of exercises can make you feel so good. **Get walking!**

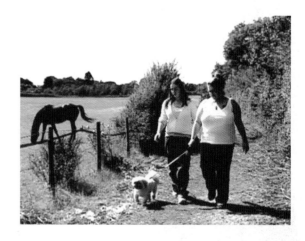

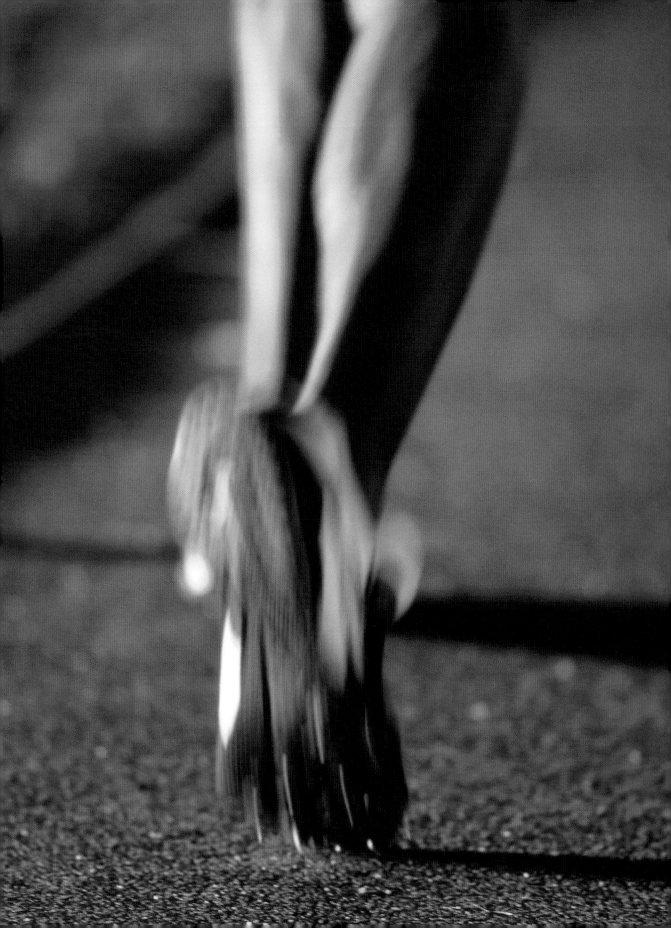

Recipes

Now that you have been given the principles of the Eating for Life food programme, and a full list of all the angel foods, we will show you some quick and easy ways to prepare these ingredients in the healthiest manner. None of the recipes require an advanced knowledge of cooking – they are all very simple to follow and virtually foolproof. As you gain experience and confidence, try varying the recipes – use different herbs and spices to see how they alter the taste of soups, stir-fries and omelettes (or Pomelettes – see page 200).

These recipes have all been prepared with sufficient ingredients to serve two people, as often recipes are designed for four – which is excessive when you are living on your own! This way, you can either have one meal today, and another cold tomorrow; or double up the ingredients if you are preparing for the family. Either way, it's easier than having to divide the ingredients or waste excess food.

Remember that the angel foods are not the only foods you should be eating, and it is important to look for new ideas every week. The major points to remember are:

+ Getting the balance right with the PCFF ratios (see page 166)
+ Portion control (see page 174)

Arm yourself with a shopping list from the Larder Essentials and the angel foods, and go shopping – it's impossible to prepare great dishes with nothing in the fridge or larder! Happy eating!

Cooking methods

Remember that olive oil is the only oil you should use for cooking. The structure of vegetable fats is altered by heating, changing them into transfats, which are potentially damaging to the body. Simply put, think of the smell that greets you when you enter a fast food restaurant – you KNOW it doesn't smell right, and the odour lingers on your clothes long after you've left the joint. That's why there is no frying or deep-frying in any of these recipes.

Where you might previously have fried a food, you can now grill it or bake it in the oven, while a food you might have deep-fried can be roasted in the oven at lower temperatures that preserve nutrients. And poaching, in water or stock, is an excellent way of maintaining flavour and succulence – Poached fish with everything in it (page 208) scores here (and, as it's cooked with the lid on, there's no lingering smell, which puts many people off cooking fish at home). In fact, one-pot cooking is a great way of combining lots of tastes into an irresistible whole – and it saves on washing up!

The recipes aren't at all complicated. Even those of you who've never really cooked a meal from scratch at home could put together any of these dishes, snacks or drinks without much fuss, although with practice you'd get to play with the flavours, and create your own versions.

They're based on two sharing, or, if you live on your own, one meal now and one later. In any case, it's generally more economical to prepare more than you need for one meal, and use up leftovers later. For example, if you're roasting a chicken, save half for cold meat, salads or a stir-fry with rice noodles, and the carcass can be used to make stock for soup. The same goes for roasting vegetables – leftovers can be puréed and added to chickpeas with cumin or turmeric and blended until smooth for a healthy low-fat dip to have with fresh, raw vegetables.

As well as making the most of leftovers, try to set aside some time in the week to prepare a few dishes and snacks in advance. That way, if you get home starving and look in the fridge for that instant fix, there'll be something to pull out – and you won't be tempted back into old snack-attack habits. You could prepare a couple of dips and store them in airtight plastic containers in the fridge, to eat with raw vegetables. Make one or two soups, and grill or bake chicken or turkey pieces (or other lean meat); store everything in the fridge when cool and keep covered. Then, when you want, simply reheat the soup, or chop up the meat for a salad or stir-fry – a matter of minutes. The time you put in beforehand is well worth the effort you save yourself when you get home.

Another tip: when you're making one-pot meals is to prepare double the quantity (or even triple), and store the remainder in the fridge for another meal the next day (or even the day after). This way you won't have to prepare every meal from scratch, but you'll be getting a selection of healthy fresh foods all the time.

The following recipes are divided into breakfasts, main meals (for either lunch or supper), snacks, puddings and drinks. The meals can all be swapped around to suit your own times and choices. The main point to remember is that you should avoid eating starches with the last meal of your day, prior to going to bed. To remind you of what these are, they include bread, rice, pasta and potatoes, but refer to page 172 for the full list so that you don't accidentally make a mistake. So, even if you're working a night shift, the meal you have before going to bed should consist of lean protein and vegetables, but no potatoes, pasta, rice or bread. This is to ensure that you don't eat excess amounts of carbohydrates before resting, as surplus amounts that are not worked off either physically or mentally will be converted to fat.

Tools for the job

Vicki says: 'There are three bits of equipment I wouldn't be without in my kitchen – a blender, a poaching pan and an omelette pan. If you don't already have these, it's worth making the investment if you can. They'll soon pay for themselves as you find it easier to prepare more of your food at home. It's a myth that fresh food is more expensive than ready-to-go – keep your shopping bills for a month and you'll be pleasantly surprised.'

+ For many of the recipes included here, a good quality blender is vital – you can make all your smoothies, dips, soups and sauces in seconds. Those with glass jugs, rather than plastic, are a better investment, as they will last far longer and you have the added advantage of being able to purée frozen fruits for smoothies or frozen stocks for soup without having to wait for them to thaw.

+ You can cook anything from fish and chicken to soups in a stainless steel poaching pan. It should be fairly shallow, flat-bottomed, and wide (about 25–30cm/10–12in round). Most importantly, it should have a heavy base to distribute the heat evenly, and a well-fitting lid to keep in all the flavours and nutrients.

+ The omelette pan is 15–18cm (6–7in) in diameter, and shallower than regular frying pans. Naturally enough, it's ideal for omelettes and other egg dishes, as well as dry-roasting any of your seeds for snacks. It should have a good quality non-stick coating so there's no need to use butter or oil.

Breakfasts
Smoothies

There are many supermarket varieties, but these tend to consist of fruits only, which raise blood sugar levels too rapidly; they can be used as part of a snack, but don't constitute a whole meal. A whole meal smoothie has each of the PCFF elements recommended in the Eating for Life food programme (see page 166):

> P – Protein, in the form of milk (either dairy, soya or nut milk) and any added nuts or seeds
>
> C – Carbohydrate, also from any nuts and seeds, plus fruit and any grain (e.g. oats)
>
> Fa – Fat (the good variety), also supplied by the nuts and seeds
>
> Fi – Fibre, also provided by the grain

The PCFF content in one tall drink! Once you've got the hang of this, you can experiment with different fruits, grains and milks/fluids to create your own concoctions.

Banana and kiwi smoothie

1 banana, roughly chopped

2 kiwis, scooped from their skins

300ml (½ pint) milk (organic dairy, soya or almond nut)

1 teaspoon mixed sunflower, pumpkin and flaxseeds

1 tablespoon live bio yogurt (optional)

+ Mix all ingredients in a blender until smooth and drink immediately, or store in an airtight container in the fridge for not more than two days.

Banana, apricot, peach and muesli smoothie

2 tablespoons nut and seed muesli (no need for dried fruits)

600ml (1 pint) milk (organic dairy, soya or almond nut)

1 banana

1 apricot

1 peach or nectarine

+ Mix the muesli and milk in a blender until nearly smooth. Add all the fruits, and continue blending until completely smooth. If the consistency is too thick, add water to the required texture.
+ Alternatively, pour the thicker mixture into ramekin dishes or tall thin glasses, and leave covered in the fridge for a delicious pudding. Don't keep for longer than a day or overnight, as the fruit will begin to ferment – causing fizziness and a change in flavour.

Warm muesli porridge

3 tablespoons
jumbo oats

2 tablespoons
rye flakes

2 tablespoons
millet flakes

1 teaspoon
pumpkin seeds

1 teaspoon
 sunflower seeds

300ml (½ pint) milk (organic
dairy, soya or almond nut)

300ml (½ pint) water

4–5 dates, de-stoned and
chopped, or 1 banana (optional)

While many people think that porridge should be made from oats, it's more interesting to
create your own mixture of grains such as rye, millet and oats to give you alternative flavours
and an increased variety of essential nutrients. If you have no alternative, use a commercially
mixed muesli, but check that there are no added sugars.

✛ Place all the ingredients except the fruit, if using, in a heavy-based pan, and leave to soak
overnight in the fridge. This allows the enzyme action to start working on the seeds and
grains, raising their protein content and creating a sweeter taste.

✛ In the morning, place the pan over a low heat, and stir until the grains have been cooked
through, but not overheated. Don't allow the porridge to boil, as this kills off much of the
nutrient content. Add the dates or banana if using, and serve. No sugar required!

Pomelette

2 eggs per person

ground black pepper

savoury or sweet seasoning to
taste (see below)

A cross between an omelette and a pancake – ideal for anyone who's used to having their
toast in the morning, but actually needs a higher protein breakfast to get their metabolism
going. You can add spices or herbs if you want a traditional omelette taste. Provençal herbs are
best, or dried sage on its own. Turmeric and ground cumin are good if you prefer something a
little spicier, or fruit purées (home-made, of course) if you tend to like something a little
sweet in the morning.

✛ Whisk the eggs until foaming on the top, with whatever seasoning you choose.
✛ Heat a small non-stick omelette pan until hot. Drop the whisked eggs into the pan and allow
them to bubble and cook until the whole of the base is set and the top of the eggs start to
cook through (this will take about 2 minutes).
✛ Using a spatula, flip the pomelette over and cook for a further 1–2 minutes. Serve
immediately. It will be completely flat, firmer than an omelette, cooked like a pancake on
both sides – and delicious!

Apple purée

2 apples, peeled and cored,
 cut in quarters

1 pinch nutmeg or cinnamon

150ml (¼ pint) water

Any fruits can be cooked, either singly or in combination, but are best simply on their own. If you want a chunky purée, cook for slightly less time, and if you prefer a completely smooth purée, you can put the cooked fruit into a blender. This purée can be stored in the fridge for up to 4 days in an airtight container.

+ Place the apples, spice and water in a heavy-bottomed pan and heat gently until the fruit starts to break down. Use a wooden spoon to stir (it won't react with the apples' acidity).

Pear and allspice purée with vanilla

2 pears, peeled and cored, cut in quarters

1 pinch allspice

2 drops vanilla essence

150ml (¼ pint) water

1 tablespoon pure organic apple juice (optional)

You could add this to the following yogurt-based recipe, or the Pomelette recipe opposite.

+ Place all the ingredients in a saucepan, and heat gently until the desired consistency is achieved. This purée tends to be tastier if left quite chunky.

Greek-style yogurt with fruit purée and toasted nuts and seeds

4–6 tablespoons Greek-style organic plain bio yogurt

2 tablespoons fruit purée or 3 tablespoons chopped fresh fruit of your choice

1 tablespoon toasted mixed nuts and seeds

+ Remember that nuts and seeds should be heated at a very low temperature to prevent their delicate essential fats from turning rancid. It's useful to make up a quantity at a time: place enough in a roasting pan to cover the base and slow-roast them in an oven heated to just 110°C/225°F/Gas ¼. After an hour they should only be slightly golden. Allow them to cool and store in an airtight container or jar until needed.

+ Put 2–3 tablespoons of yogurt in two bowls, top each with half the fruit and sprinkle with half the toasted nuts and seeds.

Basil scrambles

4 eggs

small handful of fresh basil leaves

ground black pepper

2 slices rye bread, toasted

The Italians know the lively freshness of basil and its stimulating properties – it works a treat with eggs, leaving you feeling satisfied without too full. It's great for breakfast but also good for a light evening meal after a late-night finish at work. Toasted rye bread makes a great accompaniment – Russian-style rye bread or pumpernickel are now available at all good supermarkets.

✤ Whisk the eggs until there is a light foam on the surface, then pour into a pre-heated omelette pan (a shallow pan is always best for scrambled eggs). Tear the basil leaves over the eggs as you're stirring them in the pan and season with ground black pepper to taste. Serve immediately with a slice of rye toast for maximum flavour.

Buckwheat pancakes

1 egg (or 2 eggs for a richer texture)

60ml (2 fl oz) milk (organic dairy, rice milk or oat milk)

175g (6oz) buckwheat flour (or half buckwheat and half gram flour)

Buckwheat has a more pronounced flavour than wholewheat. Some people find this too strong so, for a more subtle flavour, you may wish to combine a mixture of buckwheat and gram (chickpea) flour, using a 50/50 mix. Either way, these pancakes are packed with minerals and B vitamins, and make a great alternative to wholewheat toast for your morning breakfast – serve with chopped fruit and crème fraîche. They also make a delicious lunch, served with roasted vegetables and feta cheese. Allow two pancakes per person.

Note: You could batch-cook a larger amount and freeze the pancakes. Remember to place a small sheet of greaseproof paper in between each to prevent them from sticking when defrosting. Bag them in batches of four so you're not tempted to eat more than needed!

✤ To avoid lumps in the mixture, whisk the egg(s) first, then gradually add to the milk before adding the flour, and mixing to a smooth batter. The consistency should be that of single cream – if it's thicker, add more milk. Allow to stand for at least 15 minutes before cooking (or prepare the batter the night before, cover and leave in the fridge overnight).

✤ Heat a non-stick omelette pan until hot – test by dropping a small amount of the pancake mixture into the pan. If it sizzles, the pan is ready. Drop a small ladle of batter into the pan and roll it around to ensure a nice thin pancake. Allow to cook for 1–2 minutes before flipping it over.

✤ Cook on the second side for 1 minute then remove from the pan on to a plate. Keep finished pancakes warm in a low oven. Continue cooking until the batter is all used up.

Main meals

While these main meals are interchangeable between lunches and suppers, remember not to have starchy carbohydrates (e.g. bread, pasta, rice and potatoes) for the evening meal – they're more appropriate for lunch.

Poached fish with everything in it

1 tablespoon olive oil

1 small onion, peeled and chopped

1 thumbnail-size piece root ginger, peeled and sliced

1 orange pepper, deseeded and chopped

2 medium plum tomatoes, chopped (optional)

2 small carrots, peeled and sliced

2 tablespoons mangetout, topped and tailed

1 small head broccoli, cut into florets

2 tuna steaks, approx 2cm (³/₄in) thick

600ml (1 pint) vegetable stock

lemon or lime wedges for garnish

1 x 200g packet soba (buckwheat noodles) or rice noodles, to serve (optional)

This is one of the easiest dishes to cook, and has numerous permutations. You could start with a strong fish such as salmon or tuna steaks as these tend to keep their shape more readily than white fish, but any fish steak or rolled-up fillet will work in this case.

✢ Heat the olive oil in a large flat-bottomed saucepan, then add the onion and ginger. Sauté gently until almost transparent.

✢ Add all the other vegetables and gently stir-fry for 2–3 minutes until they are sealed. Turn up the heat a little and push the vegetables aside so you can place the tuna steaks on the bottom of the saucepan. Sauté the fish on both sides to seal.

✢ Add stock, cover tightly with a lid and allow the fish and vegetables to cook for a further 10 minutes only.

✢ Remove the lid, and serve the fish and vegetables straight into large soup bowls.

If you wish to serve with buckwheat or rice noodles, take one packet for two persons and place in the saucepan with the fish and vegetables 5 minutes before the end of cooking time. This will give the noodles enough time to be fully cooked.

Blushing swordfish steaks
with cayenne pepper on pumpkin purée

225g (8oz) pumpkin, peeled and chopped

ground black pepper

1 tablespoon olive oil, plus 1 teaspoon

2 cloves garlic, peeled and finely chopped

3 spring onions, finely chopped

2 swordfish steaks, approx 1cm (½in) thick, and 175g (6oz) each in weight

¼ teaspoon cayenne pepper

50g (2oz) French beans, trimmed

150ml (¼ pint) hot vegetable or fish stock

Swordfish is one of the meatier fish, more substantial than halibut, cod or other white fish, so buy smaller steaks.

+ Preheat the oven to 170°C/325°F/Gas 3. Rub the pumpkin cubes with the olive oil, and sprinkle with black pepper. Place on a roasting dish and cook in the oven for 30 minutes.
+ Meanwhile, put the remaining olive oil in a heavy-bottomed saucepan with the garlic and spring onions and heat through.
+ Place the swordfish steaks on top of the garlic and spring onions and sprinkle half the cayenne pepper on top of each; cook for 4–5 minutes. Turn the steaks over and sprinkle with the remaining cayenne pepper. Add the French beans and hot stock, and cover with a lid. Cook for a further 3–4 minutes.
+ While the fish is in the final stage of cooking, remove the pumpkin from the oven and mash roughly, adding a dash of black pepper and the teaspoon of olive oil.
+ To serve, put half the mash in the centre of each plate and place a swordfish steak on top with vegetables and sauce around the sides.

Note: You can cook chicken breasts in the same way or lean lamb cutlets with the fat trimmed for a more substantial meal. You can also replace the pumpkin with parsnip and sweet potato purée, using 110g (4oz) of each vegetable, according to what is in season.

Pulsing winter warmer meal-in-a-hotpot soup

1–2 tablespoons olive oil

1 medium onion, peeled and chopped

2 cloves garlic, peeled and finely chopped

1 bouquet garni, or dried rosemary, thyme and sage, or two pinches cayenne pepper and turmeric powder

ground black pepper

1.5 litres (2½ pints) vegetable stock (Marigold lo-salt stock powder for vegetarians or vegans)

PULSES – choose three from:

50g (2oz) puy (green) lentils

75g (3oz) red lentils (or split peas)

50g (2oz) chickpeas

75g (3oz) red kidney beans

75g (3oz) butter beans

50g (2oz) black-eyed beans

VEGETABLES – choose four or five from:

2 large carrots, peeled and roughly chopped

2 sticks celery, trimmed and roughly chopped

1 turnip, peeled and chopped/cubed

2 parsnips, peeled and sliced

2 red peppers, deseeded and chopped in chunks

2 yellow peppers, deseeded and chopped in chunks

1 large courgette or 2 small, washed and sliced

1 small butternut squash, peeled, deseeded and roughly chopped

2 large tomatoes, roughly chopped

1 large bulb fennel, shoots removed, and roughly chopped

Pulses are an excellent source of vegetable protein and they are also at the lowest score on the Glycaemic Index (see page 145), making them a great slow-release source of energy. The beauty of this recipe is that it is totally versatile, depending what's in your store-cupboard – a little bit of this and that and a sprinkling of herbs or spices creates a different taste every time. Be brave and experiment – you'll soon find out which flavours suit your taste-buds best. This recipe combines several, or even many, angel foods (see page 148), to give you boundless energy and plenty of antioxidant protection. Any or all of the three pulses you choose can be tinned. If you're opting for a tin of mixed beans, use up to 175g (6oz).

✤ Choose the mix of pulses and vegetables you want. Heat the olive oil in a large heavy-bottomed pan over a medium heat, then add the onion and garlic. Stir for 2–3 minutes, then add herbs or other seasoning.

✤ Stir for a further 2 minutes and then add your vegetables, the firmest first, stirring for another 4–5 minutes to lightly seal them.

✤ Add your pulses and finally the vegetable stock. Cover the pan with a lid and simmer gently for 40 minutes to 1 hour (not less, as you are using pulses and beans, which are hard to digest if not cooked through). Adjust seasoning to taste.

✤ To serve, either put it in a bowl as it is, or take the required amount of soup and blend gently until smooth. It should not be necessary to have chunks of bread with this type of soup. One or two bowls is perfectly adequate for a main meal (depending on the size of the bowl – see Portion Control, page 174).

✤ Twice cooked is best – soups and casseroles always taste better the second time around. When you've cooked your potful, leave it to cool then keep in the fridge overnight so the flavours meld together and develop further. Reheat thoroughly the next day.

Note: It should not be necessary to add salt as many of the vegetables contain natural sodium and you can increase the flavour with the herbs and other seasonings.

Light vegetable frittata

6 small new potatoes

1 medium yellow pepper, deseeded and chopped finely

50g (2oz) peas (fresh or frozen)

225g (8oz) spinach, washed and dried

1 large carrot, finely diced

4–6 baby sweetcorn, halved

1 dessertspoon olive oil

6 eggs

4–6 fresh basil leaves, or 1 teaspoon fresh tarragon leaves

ground white pepper, to taste

50g (2oz) feta cheese, crumbled

25g (1oz) shiitake mushrooms (optional)

watercress and cos lettuce salad, to serve

For those who choose not to eat eggs for breakfast but prefer them later in the day, a frittata is an excellent way of eating a bundle of vegetables together with eggs without much trouble. It's first cooked on the hob, to set the underside, then placed under a very hot grill to cook the top. This way there is no risk of breaking the omelette, as you should then allow it to cool before eating.

+ Simmer the new potatoes for 10–15 minutes until just softened. Drain and set aside.
+ Prepare the other vegetables (except the mushrooms, if using) by plunging them into boiling water, and leaving off the heat for 4 minutes before draining. Don't wash the mushrooms – just wipe off any dirt with a paper towel.
+ Heat the olive oil in a heavy-based omelette pan for 1 minute. Meanwhile, whisk the eggs together, adding herbs and white pepper as required, and pour into the heated pan.
+ Allow the eggs to settle in the pan before adding all the vegetables except the mushrooms (if using). Distribute them evenly over the whole omelette.
+ Preheat the grill. Add the feta cheese and mushrooms (if using) to the omelette, then place the pan under the grill to bubble and cook for only 3–4 minutes or until the eggs are set on top.
+ Place the pan on one side and allow to cool before removing the omelette, sliding it whole on to a similar-sized plate. Cut into quarters and serve with the salad.

Always perfect lemon chicken with six green vegetables

4 small lemons

1 medium chicken, cleaned and trussed

1 small onion, roughly chopped

4 small bok choy, washed and trimmed

50g (2oz) peas (fresh or frozen)

50g (2oz) French beans, trimmed

1 medium courgette, washed and sliced

1 small handful of watercress, washed and tied into 2 bundles

1 handful of asparagus heads (6–8), trimmed to 10cm (4in) long, tail ends removed

600ml (1 pint) chicken or vegetable stock

1 stick lemongrass (or Provençal herbs for more traditional taste)

ground black pepper

brown or basmati rice, or mashed potatoes, to serve

Marinating chicken in lemon juice gives it a great flavour. For the tastiest result, grate the zest of the lemon onto the chicken, then pot-roast it whole, along with a selection of interesting green vegetables to create another meal-in-a-pot.

✦ Grate the rind of two lemons, then cut them all into quarters. Rub the grated rind on to the chicken, place in a ceramic or earthenware casserole dish, and squeeze lemon juice all over it. Leave it to marinate in the fridge for 1 hour (or overnight).

✦ When you're ready to cook, preheat the oven to 180°C/350°F/Gas 4. Add all the vegetables and herbs to the dish, placing them carefully around the chicken, and pour over the stock.

✦ Place the dish in the preheated oven and cook for 1½ hours. Add ground black pepper to taste.

✦ Serve with the rice or mashed potatoes.

Black sesame-seed coated tofu with mixed vegetable stir-fry

1 block firm tofu

1 dessertspoon light soya sauce

2 teaspoons black sesame seeds

1 tablespoon light olive oil

2 cloves garlic, peeled and chopped

1 medium onion, peeled and finely chopped

1 thumbnail-size piece of root ginger, peeled and sliced

50g (2oz) baby sweetcorn

50g (2oz) mangetout

1 red pepper, deseeded and chopped

1 orange pepper, deseeded and chopped

300ml (½ pint) hot vegetable stock

rice or rice noodles, to serve

Tofu is a soya bean curd that is usually sold in blocks that serve two adequately. You can buy either firm or silken tofu, and the firm is best for this recipe. The beauty of stir-frying is that you simply toss the flavours in a little oil to start, and then steam the main ingredients, therefore lowering the temperature of the oil and preventing any loss of nutrients.

✦ Cut the tofu into 1cm (½in) cubes, and place in a bowl. Pour over the soya sauce and stir carefully with a wooden spoon until all the tofu is coated evenly. Then sprinkle over the black sesame seeds and ensure that all cubes are covered. Set aside.

✦ Heat the oil in a wok or frying pan and add the garlic, onion and ginger. Stir continuously for about 2 minutes, then add all the vegetables and continue stirring for another 2 minutes.

✦ Add the hot stock, top the vegetables with the tofu, and cover with a dome lid to trap the steam. Cook for a further 2–3 minutes and serve immediately with the rice or rice noodles.

recipes

Oven-roasted root vegetables

1 sweet potato, peeled and chopped

1 turnip, peeled and chopped

4 parsnips, peeled and quartered

2 red onions, peeled and quartered

1 head of garlic, not peeled, but halved

1 butternut squash, peeled, deseeded and chopped

2 tablespoons olive oil

A couple of sprigs fresh rosemary

2 sprigs fresh thyme

ground black pepper

These are a great accompaniment to a weekend roast or can be the basis for a vegetarian dish – simply add lightly toasted blanched almonds or pine nuts. The secret is to cut all the vegetables to roughly the same size, about 2–3cm (1 in) cubes, so that no one vegetable cooks much faster than the others. Don't miss out the onions – they taste great when roasted, and are vital to the overall flavour. If you have any leftovers, add them to a soup the next day or have them cold with a baked potato and chicken breast for a quick and easy lunch.

+ Preheat the oven to 175°C/350°F/Gas 4.
+ Place all the vegetables in a large flat baking or roasting dish, and baste them with the olive oil. Put the herbs over and under the vegetables.
+ Place in the oven and roast for about 45–50 minutes. Serve either hot or cold.

Brown rice risotto with spinach and pine nuts

900g (2lb) spinach

2 tablespoons pine nuts

1 tablespoon olive oil

2 cloves garlic, coarsely chopped

1 small onion, peeled and finely chopped

110g (4oz) brown rice (uncooked)

900ml (1½ pints) vegetable stock

pinch of nutmeg or allspice (optional)

This is a combination of a Spanish dish and a classic Italian dish. The Spanish tend to serve their spinach with a lot of garlic, wilting it with butter, while the Italians make risotto with sinful amounts of butter. This is a healthier option!

+ Wash and dry the spinach carefully, discarding any large and old leaves.
+ Quickly dry-roast the pine nuts in a shallow frying pan (or omelette pan) and set aside.
+ Heat the olive oil in a heavy-bottomed pan and stir in the garlic and onion until transparent.
+ Add the rice and stir for a further 2 minutes or until the rice kernels are coated and sealed.
+ Start adding the stock. The best method is to do this a ladleful at a time, stirring until all the liquid has been absorbed before adding the next ladleful. This way you won't overcook the rice. To save having to stand over the stove, you could just add all the stock in one go, stirring occasionally until it is all absorbed. The rice should be still firm (not hard), but swollen.
+ Now mix in half the spinach. When it's wilted, stir in the other half. Season with nutmeg or allspice, if using, and add a final ladle of stock to keep it moist.
+ Serve into soup plates and sprinkle with the pine nuts.

Seared fillet of beef on purée of peas with bok choy

350g (12oz) beef fillet, all fat trimmed away

2–3 dessertspoons mixed peppercorns, crushed

4 dessertspoons soy sauce

6 small or 4 medium bok choy, halved

2 dessertspoons olive oil

2 cloves garlic, peeled and chopped

500g (1lb) fresh or frozen peas

2 teaspoons olive oil (for pea purée)

Lean beef is packed with vital amino acids and is a good source of zinc for immunity and repair. Peas, while high on the Glycaemic Index, are also a rich source of antioxidants for immunity, and bok choy provides good fibre and the minerals iron and potassium. This is a high energy meal that can be served on its own, with a salad in the evening, or with brown rice at lunchtime.

+ Roll the whole fillet in the ground peppercorns and leave to stand for 10 minutes.
+ Meanwhile, heat the soy sauce in a large saucepan and place the bok choy inside face down. Allow to simmer for 4–5 minutes, then remove and place to one side.
+ Heat the oil in a pan until barely smoking, then add the chopped garlic and cook for 2 minutes, stirring gently.
+ Place the beef fillet into the pan. Roll it over until all the outside is cooked thoroughly (5–7 minutes), then cover and cook for 2 further minutes.
+ Remove from the pan and set to one side, covered with kitchen foil. (Don't discard the cooking juices, as these can be used as a sauce when serving and added to the pea purée.)
+ Meanwhile, place the peas in a saucepan and cover with freshly boiled water for 2 minutes before draining. Place immediately into a blender with the 2 teaspoons of olive oil and a small amount of the beef cooking juices to add flavour. Blend roughly (don't over-blend, as the mixture becomes too runny). Heat through again in the saucepan before serving on to plates.
+ Slice beef and arrange over the pea purée, with the bok choy around the outside. Drizzle the beef cooking juices over the meat and bok choy.

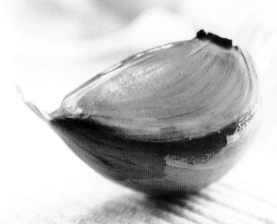

Happy snacks

Making sure your fridge is stocked with healthy snacks is possibly the most difficult adjustment to make, and yet the easiest to prepare. All you need are a couple of tins of tuna, sardines or salmon, a couple of lemons and some light crème fraîche to have an almost instant dip to eat with raw vegetables – it takes no more than two minutes! Dips and raw vegetables are the perfect mid-morning or mid-afternoon snack, with fibre and protein that give you plenty of energy.

Don't shy away from making your own dips and snacks – they taste so much better than the shop-bought varieties, and once you realise how easy they are to make, you won't buy a commercial variety again. They can be stored in an airtight container in the fridge for up to four days.

Sardine pâté

1 tin sardines in brine

1 lemon or lime

1–2 dessertspoons light crème fraîche (or plain soya yogurt for dairy-free option)

ground black pepper

pinch of paprika for added spice (optional)

+ Mash the sardines with a fork and squeeze the lemon or lime juice into the mixture. Add the crème fraîche or soya yogurt until the desired consistency has been reached.
+ Season with black pepper and paprika if using.

Smoked mackerel dip

½ teaspoon coriander seeds

1 smoked mackerel fillet

juice of 1 lemon

1 tablespoon cream cheese, or ½ block silken tofu

pepper to taste

If you have bought a double pack of smoked mackerel for a lunch and have eaten only one, use the other for a dip that is equally delicious.

+ Crush the coriander seeds in a pestle and mortar, or use a blender.
+ Mash the mackerel in a mixing bowl until chunky but not too smooth. Add lemon juice, cream cheese or silken tofu, coriander seeds and black pepper, and mix until well blended.
+ Serve with raw vegetables such as radishes, celery, endive and chicory.

Salmon spread

1 tin pink salmon in brine

1 lime

1 stick of celery or piece of
cucumber, finely chopped

1 spring onion, finely chopped

coarsely ground black pepper

2 dessertspoons crème fraîche or
½ block silken tofu

A tin of salmon can go a long way when you come home and you're starving! Dressing it up this way allows you to enjoy its rich flavour without feeling too full for dinner later – simply think of it as a luxury starter. The omega-3 oils in salmon are great for the skin so this should come into the weekly menu in one way or another.

✚ Drain the salmon and mash it. Combine with the juice of the lime, the celery or cucumber and the spring onion. Add the black pepper if desired.

✚ Mix in the crème fraîche or silken tofu until well blended. You could do this in a blender, if you want a creamy consistency.

The perfect hummus

1 large tin chickpeas, drained

2 cloves garlic, peeled

2–3 tablespoons extra virgin
olive oil

1 dessertspoon tahini (sesame
seed spread)

wholemeal pitta bread or
vegetable sticks, to serve

This is one of the least expensive snacks you can produce, costing probably a third of its commercial equivalent. It takes only minutes to prepare and offers a perfectly balanced vegetarian protein snack. It's important to combine all the flavours into a smooth dip, so using a food processor or blender will give the best consistency.

✚ Place all the ingredients with half the olive oil in a blender or food processor, and blend until smooth.

✚ Spoon into a small serving dish and make a small hollow in the centre. Pour the remaining olive oil into the hollow and serve with the pitta bread or vegetable sticks.

Home-made crisps

vegetables – any or all of beetroot, parsnip, turnip, carrots, potatoes, sweet potatoes, swede

1–2 dessertspoons light olive oil

cayenne pepper, paprika, cumin or turmeric

As a commercial packet of crisps can have a shelf-life of up to three years, it makes you wonder what else is in the packet apart from potatoes and salt! Making your own vegetable crisps is easy, and provides a much wider variety of nutrients, providing you cook them in a slow (or low-heat) oven.

+ Preheat the oven to 140°C/275°F/Gas 1. Peel the vegetables, and use a mandolin or cheese slice to slice them very thinly.
+ Rub olive oil all over a baking or roasting dish, then add the vegetable slices, moving them around so they become lightly coated with the olive oil.
+ Place the tin in the oven and cook for 35–40 minutes, turning only once.
+ When you remove the tin from the oven, drain the crisps of any excess oil on kitchen paper. Sprinkle with cayenne pepper, paprika, cumin or turmeric for flavour – do not add salt!

Homemade popcorn

1 tablespoon light olive oil

110g (4oz) popping corn kernels

cinnamon, allspice, nutmeg, cumin or ground coriander to season

Almost everyone loves popcorn, but the commercial variety is laden with preservatives to keep it crispy, so making your own is the only healthy way. And you don't have to use masses of sugar or salt for flavour – you can use cinnamon, nutmeg and allspice to sweeten it, or cumin or ground coriander for a savoury version. Experiment and see what you can come up with. Corn is packed with B vitamins for energy, and is a great source of vitamin D for healthy bones.

+ Using a heavy-based saucepan so that the popcorn doesn't burn, heat the oil and test it by dropping in one corn kernel. If it pops immediately, the oil is hot enough.
+ Pour in the remaining corn, put the lid on and hold it down while turning off the heat (to stop the oil burning). Shake the pan to allow popped corn to move to the top. When the popping stops, remove the lid and pour the popcorn into a serving dish.

Treats and puddings

There's no getting away from a sweet tooth – ten years as a nutritionist has taught me that! But there are ways of eating sweet treats more healthily. Aim to think of these as a treat, not an everyday end-of-the-meal must-have. If you need something sweet after your meal, choose a ripe peach, pear or banana.

Banana nutmeg mash

2 firm bananas

large pinch nutmeg

2 tablespoons crème fraiche, plain bio yoghurt or soya yoghurt

Not just a favourite with the kids, this usually satisfies even the most sophisticated palate!

+ Roughly mash bananas with nutmeg and half of the yoghurt.
+ Serve in bowls with remaining yoghurt spooned over top.

Mixed berry fool

2 dessertspoons mixed sunflower and pumpkin seeds (for protein)

500g (1lb) mixed berries (fresh or frozen), including blueberries

60ml (2 fl oz) water

2 dessertspoons plain bio yogurt, Oatley milk, soya or rice milk

If you eat this immediately, it makes a great breakfast smoothie. However, adding water to blueberries makes them congeal after half an hour, creating a firmer 'fool' consistency.

+ Place the mixed seeds in a blender and whiz until crushed almost to a powder.
+ Add all the remaining ingredients and blend until smooth.
+ Serve immediately for a smoothie or pour into ramekin dishes and refrigerate until set to serve as a fool.

Don't be fooled crème brûlée

4 fresh ripe apricots or 2 peaches, de-stoned and chopped

50g (2oz) brown rice, uncooked

1 vanilla pod or 4 drops vanilla essence

250ml (8 fl oz) water

1 small bio yogurt, soya yoghurt, or rice milk

2–3 teaspoons cinnamon

There isn't an ounce of cream in this dish but it does help to satisfy those creamy cravings. Easy and quick to prepare, you'd almost think it was the real thing!

+ Place the rice, fruit and vanilla pod or essence into a saucepan with the water, and cook until the rice is soft. Allow to cool slightly, then pour into a blender with the yogurt or soya/rice milk. Pulse until blended but not runny.
+ Spoon the mixture into ramekins or other ovenproof dishes. Sprinkle with cinnamon all over the top and place under a hot grill until bubbling.
+ Serve immediately or allow to cool and store in the fridge for up to 2 days.

Drinks

Endless teas, coffees and colas throughout the day are not only dehydrating, but also stressful to the body, so it's better to quench your thirst with other drinks that are beneficial.

Fruit and herb teas

Herbal teas can be included in the total amount of daily water required by the body, as they are not dehydrating fluids. However, do remember that all herbs have medicinal properties, so it is not advisable to select only one variety and drink copious cups of it throughout the day. Try several, and have no more than two cups of each variety in any one day. If you are on any prescription medication, check with your doctor if there are any herbal teas that should NOT be consumed. This is particularly important if you are taking cardiovascular or antidepressant medications, because there are several herbs that should be avoided, e.g. St. Johns' Wort, grapefruit, and artichoke. There are also a number of fruit teas that are inadvisable during pregnancy, eg. raspberry, mango, because they can induce contractions. Check with your obstetrician or preferably, a qualified herbalist or nutritionist.

Fruit teas have a tendency to store mould spores, so should not be included if you are on a yeast-free or intestinal cleansing programme because they will cause bloating and wind. Herbal teas such as artichoke and fennel are okay as they can help the cleansing process. For different benefits choose a selection from the following:

Stimulating

+ Apple and ginger (aids liver function)
+ Lemon and ginger (aids liver function)
+ Fennel (cleansing, contains phyto-oestrogens – reduces hot flushes)
+ Licorice (supports adrenal glands)
+ Ginseng and vanilla (supports adrenal glands)
+ Green tea (supports immune system)
+ Rooibosch (Red Bush) (aids digestion)
+ Nettle (supports kidneys)
+ Dandelion (stimulates production of stomach acid)
+ Echinacea (supports immune system)

Relaxing

+ Chamomile (neuro-relaxant – aids sleep)
+ Peppermint (aids digestion & reduces wind)
+ Sage (contains phyto-oestrogens – reduces hot flushes)
+ Celery seed (lowers blood pressure)

Fruit juice

Just because you are increasing your consumption of fruits and vegetables, don't think that fresh fruit juices are an easy way to increase your daily score. On the contrary, these juices simply deliver their sugars more rapidly than eating the fruits themselves, and only serve to increase your sugar cravings.

However, they should not be ruled out, because freshly squeezed or juiced fruit packs a massive nutrient punch. But do pay attention to the word FRESH. Most juices will lose their nutrient content within an hour of pressing or extracting, so ideally, you should invest in your own juicer, and make your own. If you are buying the supermarket variety, look at the sell-by date and buy only the freshest available. Remember that any carton juice that is not in the refridgerated section is not fresh, and has added citric acid and sugars to lengthen its shelf-life. These should only be consumed in diluted form, ideally no more than half juice and half water.

Juicing at home

This is an excellent way of receiving a good source of vitamins and minerals, and is generally much cheaper than supermarket varieties. You should drink your juice as soon as you have made it, to gather the maximum benefit. Don't make a large jug and store it in the fridge – only an airtight container is suitable and, even in this case, the juice should be consumed on the same day that it is extracted. The following juices are excellent for improving immunity or consuming when you are ill or low in appetite. They are best when more than one fruit or vegetable is combined.

+ Apple, ginger and watercress
+ Beetroot, apple and parsley (keep the beetroot & parsley low as they are both strong flavours)
+ Celery, spinach and apple
+ Carrot, mint and ginger
+ Lettuce, cucumber and watercress
+ Carrot, orange and mint

recipes

Why water?

It is common knowledge that we should be drinking between 2 to 3 litres water per day, but do we know why? Firstly, the human being can live for many days without food, but only 48 to 72 hours without water. Our bodies consist of 78 per cent water, which is held primarily in the intracellular fluid (the fluid that separates one cell from another), and the fluid inside every cell. There is a delicate balance of the minerals sodium and potassium that occur inside and outside the cell and that regulate the hydration of every cell in the body. When this balance is correct, all functions in the body can occur naturally, but when it is not, problems start. This is the primary reason why it is so important to drink fresh water and avoid excess salt in the diet.

Secondly, water is required to flush out the waste products that are produced naturally in the body. This is done through the kidneys, which filter all manner of fluids, and through the large intestine and bowel which deals with the digestion and elimination of all our foods (see page 60). One of the primary causes of constipation is dehydration and insufficient water intake.

Deadly dehydration

Headaches, constipation, lower back pain and lack of concentration may all be caused by dehydration. If the intracellular fluid is low, the vital nutrients that the brain and body requires for its normal functioning cannot be delivered. As a result you'll feel weak, tired and irritable. We often mistake thirst for hunger, and I always recommend drinking a glass of water as the first course of action when you feel hungry between meals. It's amazing how quickly you will perk up within minutes of drinking it. Remember that central heating, aeroplane travel and particularly air conditioning in closed offices are especially dehydrating, and you will need to drink extra water in these environments.

Which water?

Choosing bottled water has become like selecting wine – every one tastes slightly different (if you can't tell the difference between three or four types, you may be zinc deficient, since zinc is necessary for taste bud sensitivity, among many other functions). Still water is better for you than fizzy, as the carbonated waters tend to be naturally much higher in sodium. Opt for still water during the day, and save the sparkling varieties for non-alcoholic cocktails in the evening. Adding lemon or lime, cucumber batons or slices of raw root ginger all provide additional taste for those who generally don't like drinking water.

Drinking plenty of plain water is crucial for good health

If you find that drinking large amounts of water tends to increase the number of trips to the bathroom during the day, remember that this is a natural function of elimination. However, if you feel that the water is going straight through, try adding a small amount of non-citrus juice (eg apple or pear, cranberry or elderflower) as the fruit sugar molecules will help to transport the water molecules across the cell membrane – in other words, you will absorb the water more efficiently. This is not an excuse to use copious quantities of fruit squashes which are high in artificial sugars – fresh pressed juices are best.

Hydrating is better than re-hydrating

It is very important to drink water BEFORE exercising, rather than drinking to satisfy your thirst AFTER the event. Muscles will respond more rapidly and efficiently if properly hydrated, as marathon runners know only too well. Muscle weakness occurs as much from dehydration as from lack of glucose. Aim to drink approximately half a litre prior to walking, and if walking for longer than 30 minutes, take additional water with you to consume during the walk. This will prevent breathlessness and muscle cramps, especially if you have added a small amount (max 200 ml in 1.5 litres) of non-citrus juice.

As you increase the intensity of your workout, you will develop a sense of how much you need. It is not necessary to drink isotonic and other professional-level fitness drinks for moderate levels of exercise. Avoid specialised commercial 'sports' drinks which simply provide more energy through synthetic sweeteners and herbal stimulants such as guarana. While classified as natural, such herbal tonics should be avoided by those with high blood pressure, or on diuretic medications. Plain water is BEST!

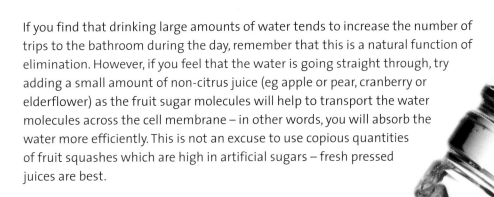

Useful websites and organisations

Testing laboratories and companies

Food allergy and intolerance home test

ImuPro UK Ltd, Unit 3, Blithfield Park Farm, Admaston, Nr Rugeley, Staffordshire WS15 3NL

www.imupro.com   01889 500 502

Food intolerance and homocysteine home test

York Laboratories, York Science Park, York YO10 5DQ

www.yorktest.com

Mineral home test kit

Nutri-Link Ltd., Nutrition House, 24 Milber Ind. Estate, Newton Abbot, Devon TQ12 4SG

www.nutri-linkltd.co.uk
www.mineraltestkit.co.uk   0870 142 0066

Pedometer with online feedback

Fitbug Pedometer   www.fitbug.co.uk   0870 228 4949

Medical organisations and societies

American College of Advancement in Medicine	www.acam.org	001 800 535 3688
The British Acupuncture Council	www.acupuncture.org.uk	020 8735 0400
British Association of Dermatologists	www.bad.org.uk	020 7383 0266
British Association of Nutritional Therapists	www.bant.org.uk	0870 606 1284
British Heart Foundation	www.bhf.org.uk	0845 070 8070
British Holistic Medical Association	www.bhma.org.uk	01273 725951
British Medical Acupuncture Society	www.medical-acupuncture.co.uk	01606 786782
The British Society for Ecological Medicine	www.ecomed.co.uk	01547 550378
British Society of Integrated Medicine	www.bsim.org.uk	
Cancer Research UK	www.cancerresearchuk.org	020 7242 0200
The Chinese Medical Institute and Register	www.chinesemedicine.org.uk	020 7388 6704

Complementary Medical Association	www.the-cma.org.uk	0845 345 5977
Diabetes UK	www.diabetes.org.uk	020 7424 1000
Digestive Disorders Foundaton	www.digestivedisorders.org.uk	020 7486 0341
The Food Standards Agency	www.food.gov.uk	
	www.eatwell.gov.uk	
Institute for Optimum Nutrition	www.ion.ac.uk	020 8877 9993
Mens' Health	www.healthofmen.org.uk	
The Prince of Wales Foundation for Integrated Health		
	www.fihealth.org.uk	020 7619 6140
The Snoring and Sleep Apnoea Association	www.britishsnoring.co.uk	01737 245638
The Stress Management Society	www.stress.org.uk	0870 199 3260
Womens' Health	www.womenshealthlondon.org.uk	0845 125 5254

Healthy eating information sources

The Soil Association	www.soilassociation.org	0117 314 5000
The Vegetarian Society	www.vegsoc.org	0161 925 2000
The Vegan Society	www.vegansociety.com	0845 458 8244
Wheat and dairy intolerance	www.wheatanddairyfree.com	
Soya products	www.sojanet.com	
Lactose intolerance	www.lactose.co.uk	
Dietary help	www.caloriecounter.co.uk	
Diabetes	www.diabetesnet.com	
Organic food	www.additive-free.co.uk	
	www.eatnatural.co.uk	01787 479123
	www.quorn.co.uk	
	www.rachelsorganic.co.uk	01970 625805
Organic food delivered to your door	www.clearspring.co.uk	020 8749 1781
	www.daylesfordorganic.com	01608 731700
	www.freshfood.co.uk	020 8749 8778
	www.organicfood.co.uk	

Height and weight conversion

From imperial to metric   www.worldwidemetric.com/measurements

1 pound = 0.454 kg   1 inch = 0.0254m
1 stone = 14 pounds = 6.356 kg   1 foot = 12 iches = 0.305m

Index

the diet doctors inside and out

index

index

Acknowledgements

With our grateful thanks to Bella Blissett for her thorough research, and Terence Barnhardt for his contribution to the fitness section; the contributors of the show, for their trust in us both, and perseverance with their individual programmes; the thousands of patients we have had in our clinics who have taught us so much over the years, and finally to the professors and colleagues who have contributed to our collective wisdom. We thank you all.

Wendy: with thanks to my patients, friends and family for their patience; Michelle and Debbie who kept my practice running while I was writing the Book. And with thanks to Robert for all of his love and support in helping me meet this challenge.

Tiger Aspect would like to thank Jamie Munro, a fair and charming deal maker, without whom this book would never have been realised; Bella Wright and Jenny Spearing for their optimism and legal insight; Amelia Dare, Dani Barry and all the *Diet Doctors* Production team for their hard work, commitment and collective talent; Matt Baker and Kathryn Flint for their unique contribution to the development of the book and promotional DVD; Sarah Sapper and Caroline Bourne for their astute financial advice; Elaine Foster, who remained calm, efficient and cheerful in the face of so many demands for photographs, stats and stills; and Paul Sommers for his wisdom and Brendan Kilcawley for his support. We would also like to thank Melanie Cantor, June Ford-Crush and Mark Wogan – honest and enabling agents all. Finally Tiger wishes to thank everyone at Ebury especially Jake, Clare, Di, Emma and Imogen for their indomitable spirit, straightforward approach and amazing 'can do' attitude – it has been a pleasure to work with you all.

The Publishers would like to thank Emma Marriott and Dan Newman for their immense professionalism and steadfast dedication to this project; Christine King for her editorial expertise; Pete Jones for photography; and Jo McGrath at Tiger Aspect, whose creative vision, support and enthusiasm kept this book on track!

Photography credits